# About the authors

**Maryon Stewart** studied preventive dentistry and nutrition at the Royal Dental Hospital in London and worked as a counsellor with nutritional doctors in England for four years. At the beginning of 1984 she set up the PMT Advisory Service which has subsequently helped thousands of women worldwide. In 1987 she launched the Women's Nutritional Advisory Service which now provides broader help to women of all ages.

Maryon Stewart is the author of the bestselling books *No More PMS!* (formerly *Beat PMS Through Diet*), now in its fourth edition, *Beat Sugar Craving* and *Healthy Parents, Healthy Baby*. She is the co-author of *The Vitality Diet*, *Beat IBS Through Diet* (now *No More IBS!*), *The PMT Cookbook* and *Every Woman's Health Guide*. She has her own weekly radio programme on health and nutrition, she has co-written several medical papers and has also appeared on several popular TV magazine shows. She has contributed regularly to 'Capital Woman', has done a series of programmes for Yorkshire TV's 'Help Yourself' programmes and has helped Anglia TV with the 'Bodyworks' series. Maryon has written her own regular page in the magazines *House and Garden* and *Healthy Eating*, and now is both advisor and contributor to *Good Health* magazine. She frequently lectures to both the public and the medical profession. She is married to Dr Alan Stewart and they live in Lewes, Sussex, with their four children.

**Dr Alan Stewart** qualified as a doctor at Guy's Hospital, London, in 1976, and spent five years specializing in hospital medicine. He is a member of the Royal College of Physicians. He worked at the British Homoeopathic Hospital in London and qualified as a Member of the Faculty of Homoeopathy. For the last 12 years he has specialized in nutritional medicine and was a founding member of the British Society for Nutritional Medicine. He is a medical advisor to the Women's Nutritional Advisory Service and is actively involved in educating other doctors on the subject of nutrition.

He is the author of several bestselling books and is the senior consultant for the Reader's Digest book, *The Healing Power of Food*. He has written medical papers and many articles in both the medical and popular press and has frequently appeared on radio and television.

Cartoons by Mik Brown

D0774497

By the same authors

*Beat the Menopause without HRT* by Maryon Stewart
*No More PMS* by Maryon Stewart
*Beat PMS Cookbook* by Maryon Stewart and Sarah Tooley
*Healthy Parents, Healthy Baby* by Maryon Stewart
*The Vitality Diet* by Maryon Stewart and Dr Alan Stewart
*Beat Sugar Craving* by Maryon Stewart
*Tired all the Time* by Dr Alan Stewart

# No More IBS!

*Maryon Stewart and Dr Alan Stewart*

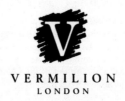

VERMILION
LONDON

First published in 1994 as *Beat IBS Through Diet*

7 9 10 8 6

Copyright © Maryon Stewart & Dr Alan Stewart 1994, 1997

The moral right of Maryon Stewart & Dr Alan Stewart
has been asserted in accordance with the Copyright,
Design and Patents Act, 1988.

First published in the United Kingdom in 1994.
This revised edition published 1997
by Vermilion an imprint of Ebury Press
Random House, 20 Vauxhall Bridge Road, London SW1V 2SA

Random House Australia (Pty) Limited
20 Alfred Street, Milsons Point, Sydney
New South Wales 2061, Australia

Random House New Zealand Limited
18 Poland Road, Glenfield
Auckland 10, New Zealand

Random House South Africa (Pty) Limited
Endulini, 5a Jubilee Road, Parktown 2193, South Africa

Random House Group Limited Reg. No. 954009
www.randomhouse.co.uk

A CIP catalogue record for this book
is available from the British Library

ISBN 0 09 181593 2

Typeset by SX Composing DTP, Rayleigh, Essex

Printed and bound in Great Britain by
Creative Print and Design Wales, Ebbw Vale

WARNING
This book gives non-specific, general advice and should
not be relied on as a substitute for proper medical
consultation. The author and publisher cannot accept
responsibility for illness arising out of the failure to seek
medical advice from a doctor.

# Contents

**Appendix**

# Acknowledgements

We would like to thank the doctors and researchers who have paved the way for us in the field of Irritable Bowel Syndrome, and whose publications have been essential to the writing of this book. In particular we are grateful to Dr John Hunter, Dr K. Wheaton, Dr P. Whorwell, and many others both in the UK and overseas.

Our sincere thanks go to all the patients who have volunteered to share their experiences and allowed us to divulge personal details about them, in the hope of helping others.

We also thank the team of dedicated workers at the Women's Nutritional Advisory Service, who make writing books a pleasant experience for us. Special thanks go to Cheryl Griffiths who helped us turn the words into a manuscript, to Allison Day who helped put the appendix together and to Clare Fitzgerald for distracting our children while we worked.

Thanks are also due to Lavinia Trevor, our agent, and to Sarah Sutton, our editor, for their professional guidance.

Finally, we would like to thank our four wonderful children, Phoebe, Chesney, Hester and Simeon for their patience, understanding and cuddles while we were burning the midnight oil.

*Maryon and Alan Stewart*

# *Miriam's story

Miriam Vince is a 33-year-old farmer's wife from Scotland. She has one child and spends part of her day being a housewife and mother and the remainder of the day helping her husband on the farm. 'Just over a year ago I had an ectopic pregnancy, which left me feeling very low. Six weeks later I contracted a bad virus infection which left me absolutely shattered. During this low period I began to experience all manner of gut problems. I would go from being constipated to having diarrhoea, sometimes in the same day, and would feel very bloated with lots of wind and abdominal pain. After bowel movements I felt very depressed and dizzy, and experienced mood and energy swings. My doctor put it all down to emotional problems, following the ectopic pregnancy, and I went along with his diagnosis.

'As the symptoms persisted I was sent to the hospital as an outpatient for a barium enema, an X-ray, and a sigmoidoscopy (looking into the lower bowel with a special telescope). As the results of all these tests were negative, I was diagnosed as having Irritable Bowel Syndrome, told to eat lots of wholemeal bread, muesli and Weetabix and I was prescribed Colofac, Colpermin, and Prozac, an anti-depressant. I was told that my symptoms might settle, but that I would always be bothered from time to time.

'The bouts of diarrhoea became so severe each morning that I would have several motions, until the bowel was empty, and then complete exhaustion hit me. After that I became frightened to leave the house. I experienced panicky nervous feelings which became worse if I pushed myself to try to be 'normal'. My doctor eventually said that I was suffering from ME (a virus causing severe fatigue) as well, and there was nothing that he could do to help.

'Luckily I read a newspaper article about the success that the Women's Nutritional Advisory Service was having using the nutritional approach to symptoms. I contacted them and subsequently took their four-month postal and telephone course. That was only three months ago, and the improvement I have achieved has been

---

* Despite the fact that most of the patients who volunteered to tell their story in the book didn't object to my using their actual names, I felt it would be more appropriate to change their names and let them remain anonymous.

great. I found that cereals, like wheat, oats, barley and rye upset my bowels, as well as caffeine. Also, milk and other dairy products seem to bring back the depression, tiredness, joint stiffness and the nasal congestion that I was experiencing before.

'I now feel as though I'm getting back to my old cheery self. I am enjoying being out and about and am at last regaining my confidence which had been well and truly crushed. Having someone who really understood the cause of my problems, who didn't think it was all in my mind, and who could guide me through on a practical level has been invaluable.'

# Introduction

For the majority of us our bowel habits are a well-kept secret. Even in these days of open communication it is not considered socially acceptable to discuss our successes or disappointments in the little room which is rarely referred to as the toilet. Our lack of ease with the subject even prevents many of us from calling the lavatory by its real name. Instead we talk about 'the loo' 'the John' 'the bathroom' or even 'the ladies' powder room', and suffer our bowel disorders in silence. Just as many of us are totally in the dark about the number of times the average couple make love each week, so too are we under-educated about what constitutes a normal bowel habit. And for even the most curious of us, the question mark usually remains over this subject, unless we run into difficulties which require medical intervention.

It is normal to break wind from our tail end at times, and yet when it happens in public it is a source of much embarrassment. Many feel comfortable telling jokes about bowel habits and there are numerous joke books written specifically to be read while on 'the throne'. However, what is not widely appreciated is that those victims of bowel disorders not only suffer with physical symptoms, their mental well-being and self-esteem also take a knock.

Many of us recognize that emotion and stress affects our gut function. Who hasn't experienced 'butterflies' or diarrhoea before an exam, a wedding or other major event in life? Those of us whose bowels settle down to a reliable and trouble-free routine once the big day has passed pay little ongoing attention to our bowels. However, individuals who continue to suffer with diarrhoea, constipation, wind, pain and bloating in the long term, often find that their bowel problem becomes all-consuming.

We know from our clinical experience over the last 14 years that bowel symptoms can undoubtedly affect our mood, our energy levels, our general well-being and the way we perceive ourselves. Being unable to control our own bowels leaves millions of people feeling like isolated physical failures. In truth, almost a quarter of the adult female population, and nearly one-fifth of men are suffering with irritable bowels, most of whom automatically believe that everyone else is symptom free. But those considerations are far from the actual situation.

Irritable Bowel Syndrome (IBS) is a label often given to an individual when members of the medical profession are baffled. The cause of IBS has confounded physicians for almost two centuries, and despite a great deal of research, no convincing explanation for it can be given. The usual sequence of medical events is that thorough investigation of bowel symptoms takes place, and when no sinister medical cause can be found, the condition is hereinafter referred to as IBS. The treatments on offer are wholly inadequate and usually consist of either taking drugs to mask the symptoms, or eating large quantities of whole wheat and bran, both of which, for many IBS sufferers, only serve to increase their suffering. Alternatively, sufferers are simply told to learn to live with it.

The notion that IBS is related to, or even caused by our psychological state is as old as the concept of IBS itself. Many studies have found that symptoms of anxiety, depression and distress are more likely to occur in patients with IBS than in people with other illnesses. However, when you consider the effect that having major gut problems is likely to have on an individual, this is hardly surprising, and although it may be an interesting theory, does not open the door to a solution.

At the Womens Nutritional Advisory Service (WNAS) we have been helping people with symptoms of IBS for over 14 years. We discovered our success in relieving IBS symptoms initially by accident, while treating women with hormonally related problems. Approximately half the patients we advise are suffering from IBS, or related conditions, and we manage to help the vast majority over their symptoms in the space of three or four months.

This book is based on our successful programme. It will allow you to conduct a controlled experiment on yourself, in order to isolate those factors in your diet that aggravate your symptoms, and thus to overcome them. Finding the right kind of diet for your body is important for your long-term health, as well as helping you to overcome the symptoms you have been recently suffering. While it may be plain sailing for some, others will find that it is a tricky business, which is why this must be a strictly controlled experiment.

The process of discovery will take ten weeks, which may sound like a long time but, in fact, is a very small percentage of your whole life. Part One of the book will give you vital information about what underlies your symptoms, will help you to identify whether there is a need for further investigation, and will tell you more about your symptoms than you have ever known before.

The diet itself is outlined in Part Two, on a day-by-day basis, with delicious menus to follow and recipes to try. For those who work we offer Fast Options, which require little preparation time and can be taken out of the house. The diet is comprehensive, without being incomprehensible, and most of all it is enjoyable. Provided nothing sinister underlies your bowel problems, it is very likely that you will be able to overcome your symptoms if you follow the recommendations closely.

Where possible, we have included case histories of patients who have been kind enough to share their stories. You will see that the vast majority of them had been suffering with IBS for a long time, and as no solution was found for them by their doctors, they were left to their own devices. After following our recommendations, they overcame their symptoms and now have a new lease of life. You could be in the same boat within a few months, just by giving the experiment outlined in this book your best shot.

Please make sure that you read Part One before you go on to the diet section in Part Two. We wish you every success and would be delighted to hear about your results, if you would like to share them with us. If you wish to write, or would like information about the clinics we hold, you will find the address of the WNAS at the back of the book.

*Maryon and Alan Stewart*

*part one*
# The problem

# 1
# IBS explained

The term Irritable Bowel Syndrome was coined in 1944 by Dr Alvarez, who suggested that physicians discard the term mucous or spastic colitis, and used the term IBS instead. He proposed that the name for the condition should include the word 'bowel' rather than 'colon', because there are reasons for believing that in some cases the small bowel and even the stomach share in the irritability. This accounts for the change in diagnosis by doctors to the term IBS, instead of spastic colon and the like, but it does not mean that they are any nearer to a workable and effective treatment to overcome symptoms in the long term.

IBS is an extremely common condition. In fact, it is so common that surveys reveal that about half of the people attending hospital out-patient departments with digestive problems are suffering from IBS. A number of specialists have suspected that the people whom they were seeing in out-patients were in fact only the tip of the IBS iceberg. In other words they thought that IBS might be a very common disorder in the population as a whole and that only a small fraction of those who suffer actually complain to their doctor.

Accordingly, several surveys have been conducted in which ordinary members of the public, not patients, were asked about their bowel habits. This has helped to give a more accurate picture of IBS and has also identified which are the most common symptoms and who gets them.

## What is a 'normal' bowel habit?

For many years the gold standard of a normal bowel habit was any frequency from three times a day to three times a week. This description of normality was obtained from a large survey conducted in the United Kingdom and published in 1965. At that time 99 per cent of the population surveyed fell within these limits. It was also discovered that many people still complain of diarrhoea or constipation because of changes in the consistency of the stool, feelings of urgency or difficult in passing a stool.

An American survey of doctors and hospital workers conducted nearly 20 years later revealed that 94.2 per cent had a stool frequency of between three times a day and three times a week. The average number of stools per week was 7.1 for women and 9.6 for men. Further questions about a variety of bowel symptoms revealed that a total of 17.1 per cent had symptoms indicative of bowel dysfunction. So much for normality.

A recent poll of nearly 2,000 patients from the Bristol area showed that many had regular bowel movements. Amazingly, only 40 per cent of men and 33 per cent of women had a regular one-a-day cycle.

Constipation was particularly more a problem for women, especially young women, with one-third of all women opening their bowels less than once a day. These recent findings are in keeping with previous ones.

## How common are the symptoms of IBS?

In the last ten years there have been several surveys looking at the frequency and pattern of bowel symptoms in different populations around the world. These surveys show relatively consistent results. IBS is common with frequencies of between ten per cent and up to 25 per cent being reported. IBS is not, for example, a condition exclusive to those eating a Western diet. A survey of bowel habits in both rural and urban-dwelling Thais revealed that five per cent had symptoms compatible with a diagnosis of IBS by standard Western criteria. Additionally, over 20 per cent complained of feelings of constipation.

A recent and detailed UK-based survey was conducted by Dr Kenneth Heaton and colleagues from the Bristol Royal Infirmary. They surveyed nearly 2,000 men and women in order to determine exactly who gets IBS and who complains about it to their general practitioner. They used a standard questionnaire that asked for many of the symptoms of IBS including the presence of the following: recurrent abdominal pain, abdominal bloating, a feeling of not having emptied the bowels properly, urgency to open the bowels, watery stools, slime in the stools, and the association of pain with any of the foregoing. The presence of three or more of these and some other bowel symptoms was taken as a positive diagnosis of IBS.

Such a diagnosis could be made in a total of 13 per cent of women aged between 25 and 69 years and in five per cent of men aged between 40 and 69 years. In women, bloating and symptoms suggestive of constipation increased with increasing age. Overall abdominal pain was the most common symptom in both men and women and affected many more women than men. Its presence was the main factor that determined whether or not sufferers of either sex had consulted their doctor. Also, the more symptoms sufferers experienced, the more likely they were to consult their doctor. So it seemed that for many with bowel symptoms their pattern of consulting behaviour was quite appropriate to their pattern of symptoms. Many, however, simply put up with their symptoms and just learn to live with them.

Similar but slightly different results have been obtained from Prof. Roger Jones and Susan Lydeard in their survey of some 2,000 adults aged 20 years and over, all of whom lived in the Southampton area. A total of 21.6 per cent (24.3 per cent of women and 18.7 per cent of men) reported symptoms consistent with a diagnosis of IBS. Not everyone in the survey completed the questionnaire, so it is possible that these figures are over-estimates. Taking this into account, the minimum total prevalence would be 15.4 per cent or two out of every 13 adults in the population. About a third of those who responded to the survey and had IBS symptoms had been to see their doctor, and less than half of these had been referred on to a hospital specialist. Diarrhoea as a complaint was more common in this group of IBS sufferers than was constipation (58 per cent compared with 48 per cent).

So no matter how you look at it, IBS is a very common condition and many of those troubled by it do not see their general practitioner or a specialist. If they all decided that they should then this would place an impossible burden upon medical care facilities in the UK.

Prof. Jones' survey also came up with many other interesting and relevant findings. The most common age group for women to experience IBS symptoms was 30 to 49 years and for men it was surprisingly 20 to 39 years. Perhaps today's young men take in too much beer and not enough fruit and vegetables. IBS was not more common among smokers and the chance of developing it did not seem influenced by social class. Also, a greater proportion of those with IBS symptoms made use of strong painkilling drugs of the sort prescribed by doctors for arthritis and used in the treatment of painful periods. These drugs are known to irritate the bowel and can cause diarrhoea. Many other common conditions appeared to be affecting those with IBS symptoms, which suggests that there may be several hidden factors that determine an individual's likelihood of developing IBS (see Chapter 3).

## What triggers IBS?

This is a very relevant question and there are a number of aspects which need to be considered.

### Age

First, it is obvious that many with IBS developed symptoms in young to middle age. However, it is also now known from Prof. Jones' survey that 12 per cent of those with IBS had experienced repeated episodes of abdominal pain in childhood compared with three per cent without IBS. So it seems that, for some, the seeds of IBS are sown in childhood or before.

### Operations

Many doctors have observed that IBS is more likely in those who have had a hysterectomy or an operation on their ovaries. Such operations may have left some internal scar tissue and this possibility should always be checked by a doctor. From one survey by Dr Prior and colleagues in Sheffield it was found that about ten per cent of women undergoing a hysterectomy developed new bowel problems in the weeks and months after their operation. Constipation with other IBS symptoms was the most common complaint. The chances of this pattern of symptoms developing was not influenced by the use of antibiotics at the time of surgery.

### Radiotherapy

Radiotherapy treatment that involves the abdomen can also trigger bowel symptoms which may persist. This could be due to irritation or scarring of the bowel itself or due to damage to the digestive function of the gut. Again, this situation requires careful assessment by a doctor.

### Gynaecological problems

The womb (medically known as the uterus) is next to the end of the colon and a significant amount of the small bowel sits loosely coiled on top of the uterus. Many conditions affecting the uterus cause the production and release of powerful chemicals which are able to influence gut function. Dr Prior and colleagues' study mentioned above also found that many of the women undergoing hysterectomy noticed an improvement in their previous bowel problems. Most of the 200 women in this study were having a hysterectomy because of very heavy periods, prolapse of the womb or enlargement of the womb due to the growth of fibroids. Twenty-two per cent of the total group had IBS symptoms before surgery and approximately two-thirds of them experienced improvement after surgery.

The simple conclusions are that gynaecological problems can underlie bowel symptoms, that some patients will indeed experience an improvement in their IBS as a result of surgery but that some may apparently be made worse or develop symptoms where none existed previously. The risk of the latter is small but definite.

## Gastrointestinal infection

Acute gastroenteritis results in sudden onset of diarrhoea sometimes accompanied by vomiting and fever. Everyone has probably experienced such tummy troubles either as children or perhaps when on holiday abroad. Most of these upsets are caused by a virus or bacteria and are expected to last between one and three days in the majority of cases. Sometimes the bowels never do settle down completely and the symptoms of IBS develop.

Inability to digest lactose (milk sugar) and a lack of vitamin B can lie behind some cases of persistent diarrhoea following an acute bout of gastroenteritis. Only a small percentage of those with IBS develop symptoms in this way.

Research from the University of Sheffield conducted by Prof. NW Read and colleagues looked at who was most likely to have persistent bowel symptoms after a bout of infectious diarrhoea. Looking at a group of patients admitted to hospital because of acute infectious diarrhoea, those who had higher scores for symptoms such as anxiety, depression and neurotic characteristics were more likely to develop persistent bowel symptoms. While this might support the notion that psychological type predisposes to IBS, some factors, such as a lack of vitamin B, which is common in those suffering from anxiety and depression, could be a linking cause for both bowel symptoms, especially persistent diarrhoea and a person's psychological state.

## Other bowel conditions

IBS can exist alongside other bowel conditions and there may be a connection between them. In older people diverticulosis of the colon (a bulging of the walls of the colon due to the weakness of its muscles) is a common condition which may exist silently or cause IBS-like symptoms. The two may have a common partial cause in a relative lack of fibre in the diet. In patients with ulcerative colitis (a severe inflammation of the colon causing diarrhoea and bleeding) symptoms of IBS can be present even when the colitis is adequately controlled by drugs. So sometimes it is important for patients with these conditions to consider the same dietary and other factors that lie behind IBS.

## Drugs

As has already been mentioned, some painkilling drugs can trigger or worsen IBS symptoms. This may happen shortly after taking them or might develop gradually after several months. Antibiotics can cause diarrhoea as a side-effect and this might set off IBS-like symptoms in some. This seems to be due to a build up in the gut of *Candida albicans*, the organism responsible for thrush. Usually such an event is self-limiting, lasting only a few days or weeks, but it has been reported as a cause of chronic bowel problems in some people.

Supplements of iron and multivitamins containing them can also irritate the gut producing diarrhoea or constipation. There are many other drugs that might aggravate IBS symptoms and these are discussed in Chapter 9.

## Stress

There is now good evidence that a variety of stress factors will worsen the symptoms of IBS. It has been shown, for example, that stress in a number of forms can cause the muscles of the bowel wall to contract in a disordered, and potentially inefficient, painful fashion. Other studies have shown that though patients with long-standing IBS, who attend hospital, may experience significant anxiety and depression, the large majority of those with IBS symptoms who mainly put up with their problems are psychologically normal. For those chronic attenders at hospital a satisfactory treatment for their IBS would go a long way to reducing their anxiety and depression. Patients with IBS are more likely to consult their doctor after a stressful life event and chronic attenders may have a history of significant stress.

## Hyperventilation or over-breathing

Over-breathing, especially rapid short breaths, results in a loss of carbon dioxide from the blood stream. This alters the acidity of the blood and body chemistry and may cause light-headedness, changes in pulse rate, tingling in the fingers, muscle cramps and weakness.

Researchers from the United States have shown that this can also affect bowel function. In an experimental situation, deliberate hyperventilation increased the level of colonic pressure as well as the episodes of contraction experienced in the first half of the large bowel. What this means is that hyperventilators or over-breathers may experience more bowel symptoms when they over-breathe, with pain being the most likely symptom to be worsened.

## A change of diet

In view of the recognized connection between IBS and intolerance to a number of foods, it seems likely that some cases of IBS are sparked off by a change in diet. This could be because of eating new foods, those which are hard to digest, or because of an increase in the amount of a particular food. However, in most of those with proven food intolerance there seemed to be no recent change in dietary habits.

## Nothing

Despite all of the above, it is very often the case that there has been no obvious single precipitating factor which starts off IBS. Perhaps it is a subtle combination of circumstances or perhaps there are hidden predisposing factors which might be genetic and therefore run in families. Doubtless future medical research will look at why some people develop IBS and others never have any problems with their bowels.

## What happens to patients with IBS?

Now for some cheering news. The first studies that looked at what happened to those with IBS gave a rather disappointing message. Two studies conducted over 25 years ago revealed that only 12 per cent and 33 per cent of the patients were recorded as having improved to the point of being symptom-free. These results were obtained before modern scientific methods allowed a clear understanding of what has gone wrong in IBS and how it can be put right.

A more recent and optimistic study revealed a symptom-free rate of 68 per cent. This group was reported by Dr Harvey and colleagues from the Frenchay Hospital in Bristol in 1987. Treatment involved a variety of approaches including a high-fibre diet, laxatives, drugs to relieve bowel spasm and, when necessary, psychotherapy and anti-depressants. Many continued with a changed diet in the long term. A number of these patients were interviewed again after five years. From this it was concluded that improvement was more likely to be obtained if the patient was male; the predominant symptom was constipation and not diarrhoea; the symptoms had been present for less than two years; if there had been some improvement within the first month of treatment, and if the IBS had been precipitated by gastroenteritis or some other illness or operation.

Women with long-standing diarrhoea seemed to do badly in this study. (Do not despair if this describes you as there are several proven effective treatments for this situation that were not part of this particular study.) The message from these findings and from our own experience is simple. There are many ways of combating IBS successfully. Do not give up hope just because one or even two or three past attempts have not borne fruit. The developments of the last decade in particular mean that, if you have to have IBS, there has probably never been a better time to have it than now!

So let us start by understanding more about the symptoms, causes and influencing factors of IBS.

# 2
# How the gut works

Now that you have read about the symptoms of IBS, and the problems that they can cause, it may help if you understand a little about how the normal, healthy bowel works. While we do not wish to bore you with science, some technical details are necessary, and are important to our understanding of IBS.

You will probably realize that IBS has, for a long time, been a poorly understood condition. Patients with it have been dismissed with the words 'there is nothing wrong with you' or 'it's all in your mind'. The reason a doctor says this is because standard tests may have not shown any problem with the structure of the bowel itself. For example, an examination, bowel X-rays or even a look inside the bowel itself are usually normal in most patients with IBS. What is wrong is not the *appearance*, shape or size of the bowel, but the *way* the bowel works. Although the anatomy or structure of the bowel is in order, its function is not. So in order to understand what can go wrong in IBS, and how it can be put right, you need to know how the normal, healthy gut works.

## What is the gut?

This may seem like an unnecessary question, but the answer may surprise you. The term 'gut' refers to any part of the gastrointestinal tract, from the mouth to the anus. Most people tend to think at first that the gut is inside the body. In fact, strictly speaking, the contents of the gut are outside the body. The gut is only 'inside' the body in the way that the middle of a ring doughnut is 'inside'. We are all actually tube shaped, and the inner aspect of our tube is what we call our 'guts'. They are a highly specialized, elongated, curiously shaped, muscular tube with a very special and important function: to obtain the nutrients essential to life from the food that we eat, and to deposit the rest.

The gut has three main components which allow it to fulfil its function: the lining, which is sometimes called the mucosa; the muscles; and the digestive glands, such as the pancreas and the liver. You may have been surprised about the comparison with a doughnut, but

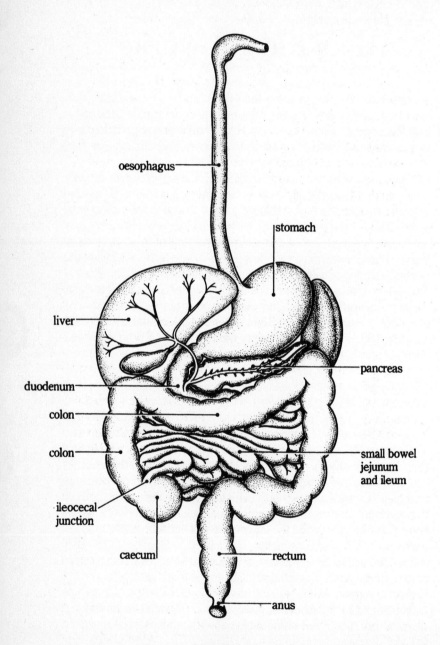

**The Gut**

it does make sense when you think about it. Really the gut is similar to skin. Both can be thought of as being on the outside of our bodies, and having the difficult task of being in close contact with a wide variety of foods, powerful digestive chemicals, bacteria, waste products and so on. No wonder they both get a little irritable at times!

The gut lining, or mucosa, lines the gut from end to end. You can see and feel it in your mouth where it is soft, moist and shiny. The mucosa is covered with a layer of cells dotted with glands that produce mucus, rather similar to the watery catarrh you get when you have a cold. This lining has to stop undigested food from entering into the bloodstream but allow the digested sugars, fats, proteins, vitamins and minerals to pass through. In IBS this lining is normally quite healthy. Occasionally it can be damaged if there is a lack of vitamin B or iron and it is often inflamed or ulcerated in conditions such as colitis or Crohn's disease.

The next part is the muscles of the bowel. There are two layers of muscle that extend from the throat, and are involved in all the processes, from swallowing, right the way through to the muscles at the end part of the bowel, in the rectum and anus, which are used when we go to the toilet. They all work to propel food through the gut while it is being broken down, digested, and absorbed into the body, and while the waste residues are formed. This whole process normally takes between one and two days in most men and up to three days in women. This is the theory of what should happen with a healthy gut.

In those with IBS, the muscles of the gut can either be overactive, underactive, or they can contract in an inefficient or uncoordinated fashion. These muscles are not directly under our control in the way that arm or leg muscles are. Instead, they contract and relax in a careful, systematic fashion influenced by the digestive events in the bowel as well as other factors. The two layers of muscle are arranged in opposing fashion. One stretches around the bowel so that when it contracts a tight ring forms around the bowel. The other layer stretches along the bowel, so that when it contracts a wave of contraction can pass along it.

In order for food and digestive material to pass smoothly along the bowel, both muscle layers must work together in a carefully coordinated fashion. First, the ring muscles, which are found at the entrance or exit to the stomach, must relax. This is then followed by a wave of muscular contraction which pushes a ball of food along the gut and slowly progresses down its length. Thus there is a wave of muscle activity passing along the gut carrying with it the contents of that part of the bowel. Each muscle contraction is preceded by an area of muscle relaxation before it. The high pressure generated by the bowel contraction pushes the bowel contents forwards into the low pressure area of the relaxed bowel.

It appears that in some people with IBS this smooth co-ordinated wave of relaxation and contraction does not happen. As a result the pressure and pain build up if a wave of contraction meets a part of the bowel that is not relaxed, or which is actively contracting itself.

## The ileocecal junction

Pain in the right-hand lower portion of the abdomen is a common symptom in IBS. Pain in this area can also occur in appendicitis or ovarian problems in women. Naturopaths and other complementary practitioners often describe it as spasm of the 'ileocecal valve'. The ileum is the last part of the small bowel, the end of which joins on to the side of the first part of the large bowel, the caecum.

Some of the muscles of the caecum are arranged so that they contract in a semi-circular or circular fashion to act as a valve. Conventional anatomy texts assign little importance to this ileocecal valve, but recent research suggests that it does exist but that there is significant variation in it from person to person. In a recent Italian study, the contraction of this valve can be seen on telescopic examination in approximately 50 per cent of patients. Furthermore, examination of these tissues under the microscope shows that there are arrangements of the muscles in a circular fashion. It would seem likely from other work that these muscles can indeed go into spasm as a result of possible food intolerances, a lack of fibre in the diet or stress.

This is a small but important discovery that helps to explain patients' symptoms and allows us to understand that the observations of non-medical practitioners were probably quite valid.

## What has gone wrong?

The two layers of gut muscle are connected by a fine network of nerves which co-ordinate their actions. However this also allows the bowels to be influenced by stress through the connection to the nervous system. Additionally, it seems likely that the muscles in the wall of the bowel can be stimulated by the local effect of a food or other substance present in the bowel. This is in fact how many laxatives work including those that are derived from plants such as senna or cascara. Indeed many of the symptoms of IBS can be explained as a disturbance in the smooth functioning of these muscles that form the gut wall. They appear to have become over-sensitive to certain foods or other factors that can disturb the normal and regular waves of muscle activity that pass along the gut.

Finally, we should mention the digestive juices which are produced by the stomach, the liver, the pancreas gland and the small glands in the wall of the small bowel. These are not usually disturbed in the majority of those with IBS and so weight loss and severe nutritional problems are uncommon in IBS. Occasionally a problem in the digestion of certain types of food produces symptoms which are so similar to IBS that they are virtually indistinguishable.

## *What else goes on in the gut?*

There are several other very important components to the gut and to its activities. The gut is not just muscle and mucosa lining. Between these two layers, and elsewhere in the gut, there are millions of blood vessels, large and small, like the roots of a tree. One of their main functions is to provide oxygen to the busy muscles of the gut, and also to carry digested food, including the vitamins and minerals, around the body, particularly to the liver. As a result of this, there is an even distribution of whatever you eat throughout the body.

The bloodstream also carries with it many white cells that are constantly on the look out for uninvited guests, such as bacteria or other germs. These blood cells come into action if there is an attack of gastroenteritis, infection with a parasite or an ulcer, for example. They are also important if anything else causes irritation to the bowel lining, and sometimes it appears to be food.

The white cells, often for reasons which cannot yet be satisfactorily explained, can release a variety of chemicals in response to a food to which a person's body appears to be intolerant. These chemicals are the same as those that are released when there is physical injury or infection in the body. Their presence results in pain, swelling and a disturbance in the function of that part of the body. In the case of the bowel, the effect seems mainly to disturb the way in which the muscles of the bowel work. Sometimes these changes in the immune system of the bowel occur as part of a widespread and severe allergic reaction, as can happen in some people with eczema or arthritis.

Another important element of the normal bowel is the inhabitants that live especially in the large part of the bowel. Here food has finished being digested and absorbed and is simply waiting to be passed out as faeces. A little water is absorbed and perhaps a few minerals but not in any great amount. The material that leaves the small bowel and enters the large bowel or colon is composed of food residues that are largely indigestible by our systems. They are however of interest to the billions of friendly, and at times not so friendly, bacteria that inhabit the dark, moist, warm, oxygenless world known as your colon! In fact there are more bugs in your gut than there are cells in the body. Fortunately they are composed of a substantial majority of harmless, friendly bacteria, whose main function in life is to break down the fibrous remains of your last meal. In the process a small amount of energy is released and varying amounts of gas and sometimes acids are also produced.

A change in the type of bacteria in the bowel does seem to be important in some people's IBS. The welfare of these bugs, good and bad, is influenced by many factors including our diets, how good our digestion is, our alcohol consumption, whether we have recently taken a course of antibiotics, and food intolerances of which we may or may not be aware. All these factors need to be taken into account when looking for the cause of IBS.

Well that's enough about the way in which the normal gut functions. Hopefully you are now beginning to appreciate what can go wrong in IBS. Armed with this information, it should be easier to work out what may lie behind your IBS symptoms.

# The symptoms of Irritable Bowel Syndrome

In this chapter we are going to look at the different symptoms of IBS and how they are produced. By now, from the previous chapters you should have a reasonable idea of how the bowel and gut work and how things can go wrong. So let's take a look at the symptoms of IBS. The main ones include:

- Constipation – opening the bowels infrequently or hard stools.
- Diarrhoea – loose rather than just frequent stools.
- Alternating diarrhoea and constipation.
- Abdominal discomfort or pain.
- Abdominal bloating.
- Excessive wind.
- Mucus or slime in the stool.
- Nausea and loss of appetite.
- Indigestion.

Numerous other varied symptoms not related to digestion.

As a rule there will always be either diarrhoea or constipation (or a combination of the two) together with abdominal bloating and some discomfort or pain. These are the most common typical symptoms. Other symptoms, many of which do not relate to the bowels, may or may not be present, and may determine whether there is any other problem. These symptoms often begin gradually and for many are not severe though they can be troublesome. For these and other reasons, many with IBS have endured their symptoms for years before mentioning them to their doctor or doing anything about them.

Let's look at these different symptoms in turn and try to explain what is actually going on.

## *Constipation*

Here quite simply the bowel is sluggish, and therefore not doing its job properly. This could be due to the colon being understimulated by a lack of fibre in the diet, a lazy bowel muscle which does not contract regularly and strongly, or bowel muscles that when they do contract do so in a poorly co-ordinated fashion.

Constipation is more common in women with IBS than in men with the same condition, and in fact women without IBS often have a more sluggish bowel movement than men. In patients with IBS, constipation is often accompanied by straining when going to the toilet and no sense of satisfaction after attempting to empty the bowel. Severe constipation is sometimes a problem in young women who may also have hormonal and gynaecological problems, and as this is such an important area we have covered it in some detail in Chapter 5 (see page 28).

## Diarrhoea

This means loose stools which usually occur because food has passed too rapidly through the stomach, into the small bowel and then through the colon. This happens in some with IBS and can be accompanied by abdominal cramps and muscle contractions. Other sufferers, however, have painless diarrhoea and, when this is the case, there seems to be relatively little bowel muscle activity. The diarrhoea can therefore be due to over-sensitive bowel muscles or due to the contents of the bowel irritating the gut in some way.

Diarrhoea should be distinguished from a need to go to the toilet frequently to pass a normal stool and from urgency – which is when people have a *sudden* need to go to the toilet. The type of stool, rather than the frequency with which stools are passed, gives a guide to how quickly food moves through the gut. In healthy men and women, this journey from one end to the other usually takes anything from 24 to 60 hours. In IBS a loose stool that can be described as being 'mushy, or composed of soft blobs or just watery' is likely to have taken less than 24 hours to make the journey. A stool that can be described as 'separate hard lumps, like nuts or sausage-shaped but lumpy' is likely to have been on a go-slow and taken 60 hours or more. Diarrhoea, if prolonged, could lead to a lack of some nutrients but this rarely, if ever, occurs in IBS.

## Alternating diarrhoea and constipation

This combination is surprisingly common and suggests that there is a marked disruption in the normal smooth functioning of the bowel muscles. It can often be caused by a variety of dietary factors, stress and sometimes other medical problems.

## Abdominal pain or discomfort

This is one of the most common symptoms for many IBS sufferers, though some people have no discomfort at all. The pain can be almost anywhere in the abdomen from just under the ribs to very low down. The most normal sites for the pain are on the right or left sides in the lower part of the abdomen. Sometimes the pain extends across the whole of the lower half of the abdomen, and backache can accompany the abdominal pain.

Severe pain or tenderness in the abdomen should prompt your doctor to consider other possible digestive problems. However, it can be due to IBS. Often the pain is accompanied by a need to open the bowels and is likely to be due to a contraction of the colon muscles which are pushing along a stool ready for expulsion. Patients with IBS are actually more sensitive to a build up of pressure in the bowel than are non-sufferers.

It has been shown that those with painful constipation are likely to have high pressure, and frequent, bowel muscle contractions that are not very effective in propelling food and waste material along the bowel.

## Abdominal bloating

This is another common symptom. It is often due to a build up of wind or a sluggish and constipated bowel, though fluid retention and lax abdominal muscles can also contribute to this symptom. The bloating may be painful or painless, and often results in the sufferer having a lower self-image because very often clothes don't fit. Abdominal bloating is best tackled by addressing the underlying problems of bowel sluggishness and anything that can influence wind production.

## Excessive wind

Time for a few home truths. Everyone makes and passes wind, though some do so more than others. The average amount is apparently about 1½ litres of gas per day – enough to fill a small balloon. Over the course of a year this adds up to about 500 litres.

Gas in the bowel can come from either the air that we swallow with our food, or that which is made during the course of digestion. The amount of air that is swallowed is usually not very great and much of it is absorbed during the course of digestion or brought back

up by burping. Most of the wind that we pass is produced by the
action of bacteria in the colon breaking down residues of food in the
same way that yeast breaks down sugar to make alcohol, and produces gas in champagne.

The wind in the bowel is made up of a variety of different gases including carbon dioxide, methane (a gas peculiar to bacteria) and
hydrogen sulphide (which smells like bad eggs). The production of
these gases is complex and influenced by both diet and digestion.
For both the interested and the afflicted, we have covered this subject in more detail in Chapter 8.

## Nausea and indigestion

Nausea, a poor appetite and indigestion are symptoms that signify
that there is something awry with the upper part of the gut. Indeed,
it is now known that a disturbance in the function of the muscles of
the oesophagus (gullet) and stomach can all be part of IBS, and again
may also be affected by stress and the type of diet we eat, especially
the amount of tea, coffee and alcohol we consume as well as the
overall balance of our meals.

These symptoms are not as common as abdominal bloating, constipation and diarrhoea. If they are present without the symptoms of
lower bowel disturbance then they may well be due to some other
problem such as excess acid in the stomach or an ulcer. These possibilities require careful consideration because their treatment is very
different from that of IBS.

## Slime or blood in the stool

These symptoms suggest that there is some irritation of the colon or
lower bowel. Bleeding should only ever be slight and all bleeding
should be investigated further by your doctor or specialist. Slime, or
mucus as it is also known, is simply catarrh produced by the glands in
the lining of the bowel which have become irritated. While these
symptoms do not occur in all patients, they are not uncommon.

## Other symptoms

This section is worthy of a book in itself. For many years IBS was
seen in isolation as a digestive or purely a bowel problem. This is not
the case. Many doctors have observed that a wide range of both
physical and mental symptoms are more common in those troubled

by IBS than might be expected. Their presence or absence does not make any difference to the diagnosis of IBS, but can alter the treatment of it. Common accompanying symptoms include fatigue, migraine headaches, flushing, palpitations, backache, urinary problems, pain on sexual intercourse, bad breath or an unpleasant taste in the mouth, and vomiting. Not all these other symptoms are due to bowel or digestive problems. Certain groups of symptoms tend to be found together, and it may be that some types of people, who perhaps are more likely to get IBS, are also likely to develop other minor health problems.

Additionally, some of the factors that cause IBS can also cause some of the above symptoms as well, so there may be a common thread. It is a mistake to assume that the presence of these other symptoms should be used as evidence that the sufferer is in some way mentally unstable, over-sensitive or depressed. Since many of these less obvious symptoms cause a great deal of stress to the sufferer, we mention them again in the treatment section of the book.

# Diagnosing IBS

Finally, it is necessary to explain how doctors use the above symptoms and other information to diagnose IBS. Twenty years ago the approach to IBS was one where abdominal symptoms were assessed with a view to diagnosing a stomach or duodenal ulcer, gall stones, digestive problems or troubles with the colon or large bowel, especially diverticulosis. IBS was a diagnosis made by the doctor only when nothing else could be diagnosed. This meant that a lot of patients were subjected to a number of investigations, such as blood tests and X-rays that weren't always necessary. Consequently the end result was often unsatisfactory for patient and doctor alike, with the patient being dismissed from the surgery or hospital with little in the way of treatment except the reassurance that 'there is nothing seriously wrong with you'.

Times have changed. It has now become apparent that IBS is often the most likely diagnosis for many young to middle-aged patients with abdominal pain or a disturbance in their bowel habits. Furthermore the cost, inconvenience and also health risk of investigating the majority of patients for all of the problems mentioned above were considerable. So it had to be possible to make a diagnosis of IBS in many patients without subjecting them to a long series of investigations. As there are no tests that allow doctors to be absolutely positive about the diagnosis, it is often made on a balance of probabilities, depending upon the type of symptoms, their severity and the factors that make them better or worse.

It has recently been suggested by a group of experts that there are a set of symptoms that can be used to make a positive diagnosis of IBS, with a good degree of reliability, in most cases. The five experts, Doctors Thompson, Creed, Drossman, Heaton and Mazzacca established the Rome criteria which are continuous or recurrent symptoms for at least three months of abdominal pain or discomfort which is

- relieved by defaecation
- and/or associated with a change in the frequency of stools
- and/or associated with a change in the consistency of stools

plus two or more of the following, at least a quarter of occasions or days

- more than three stools per day or less than three per week
- altered stool form (lumpy/hard or loose/watery)
- altered stool passage (straining, urgency or feeling of incomplete evacuation)
- passage of mucus
- bloating or feeling of abdominal distension.

In other words, a doctor can be fairly certain of making a diagnosis of IBS if this pattern of symptoms is present, if there are no other major symptoms and if physical examination is normal. So it is most important that your doctor asks you carefully about your symptoms and has the time to examine you as well.

# 4

# Sinister symptoms

It is essential that we mention some of the possible conditions and symptoms that are similar to IBS and may be mistaken for it. Some of these conditions, in particular, should be considered because their treatments can be very different from those that are successfully used for IBS. Here is a check-list that may help you to decide whether you have problems other than IBS. *Remember that neither these questions nor this book are substitutes for a thorough assessment by your own doctor. If any of your answers to the following questions are positive, you should arrange a check-up with your doctor to talk about your symptoms.*

## *Check-list*

1 **Have you only recently developed symptoms which are severe?** In this case it is always best to check with your doctor if you have not already done so.
2 **Do you have severe abdominal pain?** For example, can it wake you from your sleep? Does it cause you to stop what you are doing? Does it put you off eating?
3 **Have you lost weight because of your bowel problems?** Losing anything more than a few pounds in weight should not be regarded as part of IBS.
4 **Do you regularly pass more than four stools a day?** Diarrhoea from any cause can contribute to a loss of essential nutrients, even if there is no loss of weight.
5 **Have you passed blood in the stool or passed a dark-coloured stool?** Loss of blood from the bowel requires investigation because it may not always be due to IBS.
6 **Have you had a fever with your bowel symptoms?** Infection in the bowel from parasites or other causes should be considered. Some parasitic infections can be found in the UK without travelling abroad.
7 **Have you had any abdominal operation including appendicectomy?** Past operations can leave strands of tissue called adhesions that can interfere with normal bowel function. If you have bowel symptoms and any history of operations on

the bowel or abdomen, then it is best to see your doctor.

8 **Are you aged 50 years or more?** This increases the risk of bowel problems being due to cancer or a polyp (a small growth inside the bowel) which may become cancerous. Again, you should check with your doctor if you have not already done so.

9 **Did your mother, father, sister or brother develop cancer of the bowel under the age of 50?** If so, you should also check with your doctor. Sometimes this type of problem can run in families affecting relatively young or middle-aged members. Early detection of those at risk is now possible with a marked improvement in outlook for them.

## For women

10 **Do you have any vaginal discharge, pain on intercourse or pain very low down in the abdomen?** Infection of the Fallopian tubes is particularly common in young women with these symptoms, which may sometimes aggravate or be confused with bowel symptoms.

11 **Are your periods painful, heavy or irregular?** A number of gynaecological problems may cloud the picture at times. Fibroid growths on the womb, cysts on the ovaries and sometimes hormonal problems should all be considered if you have any of the above.

## —————————— Dick's story ——————————

Dick first noticed abdominal bloating and wind when he was in a stressful job as a city accountant. Hurried meals, long hours and a diet with many convenience foods did not suit his digestion. Having a bran-based breakfast cereal was his answer to the problem but it was not a very satisfactory one.

The solution was relatively straightforward and involved him substituting his cereal for one containing oats, eating more fruit and vegetables, avoiding certain foods that increased the production of wind and eating under less stressed circumstances.

All was well for three years when his symptoms gradually returned although there had been no change in his diet or work circumstances. He still looked a healthy 58 years and examination was reassuringly normal. It seemed appropriate to try him on a fairly strict exclusion diet similar to the one that he originally followed and that had resulted in him making the original changes to his diet. The only point of concern was that he had noticed a small amount of blood in the stool on two occasions in the previous few weeks. He had been troubled by piles in years past and put it down to that. It was explained to him that unless he was completely better within ten days on the diet then he would need further investigation and certainly if he passed blood again.

As it turned out, he bled quite heavily the next week and was admitted to hospital as an emergency. He had an early cancer of the colon which was successfully removed by the surgeon and resulted in complete clearance of his bowel symptoms.

## Rosemary's story

Rosemary was a 30-year-old travelling representative who had been diagnosed with ulcerative colitis three years earlier. Treatment with drugs including steroids had been quite successful in controlling the pain and bleeding that had troubled her at the outset. However, she was still left with diarrhoea up to six times a day even when taking the drug Lomotil to control it. The diarrhoea and urgent need to go to the toilet made her work very difficult and her journeys had to be planned with great care. Surprisingly despite these bowel problems she had never lost weight from a steady 95 kg (15 stone). The diarrhoea was troublesome enough for her surgeon to consider operating to remove the colon.

The persistence of her diarrhoea without bleeding, pain or loss of weight suggested that her colitis was perhaps no longer the main problem but that she might have associated IBS. A weight-reducing diet that excluded foods commonly associated with IBS was called for and so she followed our Vitality Diet with a few modifications. This is a diet we devised to help individuals find the right kind of diet for their body.

Progress was slow and steady. After a month her weight had fallen by several pounds and her diarrhoea was better controlled though she still needed a fair amount of Lomotil. After six months her weight was down to just over 70 kg (11 stones), she had stopped taking Lomotil and the dosage of the other drugs she took to control the colitis was also reducing. Adding back certain foods seemed to aggravate the abdominal pains, particularly when she ate potatoes and white bread.

Just when we thought that the worst was over for her, Rosemary developed severe intermittent pains in the right upper part of the abdomen. These pains lasted two or three hours at a time and were associated with her stools being paler in colour. This sounded very much like the symptoms of having gall stones. Investigation by her surgeon confirmed this and they were removed by an operation.

It is important to remember that IBS is common and can coexist with other bowel conditions producing similar symptoms. Usually the pattern of symptoms gives a good idea of what the problem is.

So much for the rather sinister side of symptoms. Do not worry if you answered 'Yes' to one or more of the questions above. You now know what you should do. Your doctor may need to examine you, arrange for some tests or ask you to see a hospital specialist. The important thing is for doctors, when assessing patients with possible IBS, to be thorough. In this way those who are likely to respond to dietary treatments can be identified and those who have other problems do not waste their time and trouble with the wrong approach. That said, your doctor may say that it is perfectly all right for you to follow one of the diets in this book, even if you need to have some tests done as well.

# Constipation and IBS

## Brenda's story

Brenda Crean is a 34-year-old housewife with two children, and lives in Sussex. When she came to the clinic she had been suffering with severe bowel symptoms for years, and had extreme PMS.

'I was at my wits' end when I read about the Women's Nutritional Advisory Service. I had never felt so ill, the quality of my life was not worth talking about, and my marriage was on the rocks. I spent most of my life in pain, suffering with severe constipation, abdominal bloating and pain and awful wind. I also had dreadful PMS for two weeks a month, which made things even worse. I felt withdrawn, aggressive and would "see" little people out of the corner of my eyes. I felt exhausted all the time, I couldn't cope with the children and I seriously thought that I was going insane.

'I had visited my doctor on numerous occasions, but he was at a loss to know what to do with me. He prescribed Fybogel, strong painkillers and anti-depressants, and suggested I eat bran and other high-fibre grain products. He told me that I would have to learn to live with my symptoms.

'Through the WNAS I found that high-fibre cereals, bread and pasta, wine, coffee, caffeinated tea and chocolate biscuits were aggravating my symptoms. I followed the diet rigidly, took the vitamin and mineral supplement Optivite for my PMS, and did three sessions of exercise a week. All my symptoms disappeared over a period of three months. I just couldn't believe it could be so simple. In fact I felt so well, that I became complacent, and gradually went back to my old ways of eating. My symptoms came back with a vengeance and I felt like I was back to square one!

'I feel that I have benefited enormously from the education and guidance I have received from the clinic because I now know what upsets my bowel. Occasionally, I go "off the rails", but I know how to get back to feeling well again.'

Though there are many jokes and amusing images associated with constipation, those who suffer, or who have suffered, with severe constipation know how badly it can affect their health and their general well-being.

Mild constipation is a common affliction of those living in industrialized countries. A change in lifestyle and a relatively poor intake of fibre-rich foods are thought by many to be important in the development of appendicitis, gall stones, cancer of the colon, varicose veins, heart disease and diabetes. This much is now quite well known. What many of us may not be aware of is that other disturbing health problems are also associated with severe constipation in young women. These include:

- Breast lumps and pre-cancerous changes in breast tissue.
- Hormonal abnormalities – a low oestrogen level.
- More painful and irregular periods.
- A greater chance of hysterectomy or operation for a cyst on the ovary.
- Pain on intercourse and difficulty achieving an orgasm.
- Infertility.
- Hesitancy in starting to pass water.
- Cold hands and a tendency to faint.

Curiously the group of women who suffer with these problems do not tend to eat less fibre than others, nor are they mentally ill, but they may have experienced more stress in the past.

These diverse health problems can mostly be explained by two changes in the body that are known to exist in those troubled by severe constipation.

First, the bowel plays an important part in the metabolism of oestrogen, the female sex hormone. After it has been produced by the ovary, oestrogen passes to the liver which removes it from the blood circulation, changes it into an inactive form, and passes it out in the bile. It has now reached the digestive system, but that is not the end of the story. Once in the bowel, some of the inert oestrogen is converted back into an active form by the bacteria in the colon and is then reabsorbed into the bloodstream. Other bacteria may break down the oestrogen so that there is little useful hormone to be reabsorbed. So the type of bugs in the bowel and how quickly or slowly the bowels work can have an influence on female hormone metabolism.

Secondly, many of these women appear to have poorly co-ordinated and excessive contraction of the muscles around the lower end of the bowel and elsewhere. The muscles of the pelvic floor are the muscles that we almost unconsciously relax when we sit down to open our bowels and that we tighten when we have finished. You can feel them tighten when you pull in your tummy muscles and draw up your buttocks together as though you were trying to stop yourself peeing half way through. In women with severe constipation these muscles are often tensed and do not relax easily when there is an urge to open the bowels. For some the subsequent rise in pressure can be painful. These same pelvic floor muscles also surround the urethra which lets urine pass from the bladder to the outside world so it is not surprising that there can be a delay in the passing of urine too. Finally, the walls of the vagina are also supported by these pelvic muscles and if they are tight then intercourse may well be painful.

## Wanda's story

Wanda was a 45-year-old cabaret artist in a London night club. Maintaining her health and appearance were vital to her, and because of her many health problems she had a love-hate relationship with the medical profession.

As well as IBS she also had an underactive thyroid, depression, fatigue, premenstrual anxiety and a number of personal stresses. There always seemed to be something wrong despite her having seen many specialists. Her main bowel symptoms were severe constipation, bloating and wind. Only rarely did she experience diarrhoea.

Over many months of dietary trial and error her bowel habit became much more regular. She was helped by regularly taking a bulk laxative of psyllium husks (a rich source of fibre derived from tropical plants), eating plenty of fruit and vegetables, and avoiding most wheat, oats, barley and rye – though she could tolerate the occasional piece of white bread. She also took regular physical exercise, and supplements of magnesium and multivitamins on a daily basis, since blood tests had revealed that her blood magnesium was low. She was also almost able to stop her previous excessive use of senna-based laxatives. Her thyroid specialist needed to make a careful adjustment to her dosage of thyroid hormones and eventually she had to take Hormone Replacement Therapy pills though the progesterone component of this could aggravate her constipation.

Wanda is an all too good example of how severe long-standing constipation and IBS can be associated with a wide range of physical and mental symptoms. When her bowel was controlled she felt very much better both physically and mentally and was able to experience the proper benefit from her hormone therapies. Avoiding excessive use of senna and controlling her constipation by these other means was vital as continuing on high doses of laxatives could have led to permanent damage to the large bowel nerves and muscles and even worse constipation.

---

Much of these important findings about constipation and other health problems have only become apparent during the last ten years thanks largely to the pioneering work of Prof. Lennard-Jones and colleagues at St Mark's hospital in London. In 1986 a leading article in *The Lancet* medical journal commented that 'Severe constipation in young women is a serious, common, but neglected condition . . . '. Severe constipation is defined by most doctors as only opening the bowels twice a week or less and, as a rule, then only with the help of laxatives.

Most women with IBS and constipation are not so severely affected but there is a considerable overlap between the two groups. Men with IBS can also have difficulty in opening their bowels because of a lack of co-ordinated and appropriate contraction and relaxation of their pelvic and bowel muscles. Some of these have constipation and others have diarrhoea and constipation. Women with IBS are also more likely to have pain on sexual intercourse as well as a wide variety of other gynaecological and health problems. So, for many IBS sufferers, constipation is the most evident symptom, but by no means their only problem.

# Causes of constipation

Now, let's look at some of the causes of constipation, and particularly how they relate to IBS.

## *Lack of fibre*

Until the early 1970s IBS was commonly considered to be best treated by a low roughage (vegetable fibre) diet. Then came the observations of Dr Painter, a British Naval surgeon, who noticed the association between a high fibre intake and an absence from many of the diseases of civilization. IBS was one of these diseases of the modern world, and he thought that a lack of fibre might perhaps be its cause. A number of experts have recommended that the UK population as a whole should increase its fibre intake by about 40 per cent. This means that everyone should eat on average about 40 per cent more fruit, vegetables and cereals (bread and other foods containing wheat, oats, barley, rye and sweet corn – maize).

It has since been shown in a number of situations that the larger the intake of dietary fibre the larger is the resultant output of stool. The larger the output of stool the quicker is the passage of food from one end to another – this is known as the 'gut transmit time'. However, not everyone's body conforms to these simple rules. Girls' bowels move more slowly than boys' and some girls have very slow bowels despite a reasonable fibre intake. So, though increasing fibre intake always increases the weight of the stool, the effect of this can be quite variable and, as you may already know, more fibre is not always the answer to constipation and IBS.

## Wheat and other grains

One of the first trials of wheat bran, a rich source of dietary fibre, in IBS was conducted by a group of doctors from Bristol Royal Infirmary and the results appeared in *The Lancet* medical journal in 1977. Six weeks of a diet high in wheat fibre was reported as being of significant benefit in that it helped to increase the frequency of bowel movements, reduce the pain and the amount of mucus in the stool, and also reduce the number of contractions by the colon muscles. Curiously these doctors used Allinson's bran. Allinson was a 19th-century doctor who was struck off the medical register for advocating the health benefit of wholemeal as opposed to white bread.

These results were true for the group as a whole, but within the group studied it could be seen that for some having extra fibre in the form of 20 g (¾ oz) fine unprocessed bran was actually of no benefit, and two of the twelve patients reported that their pain was made worse.

Many studies followed and the overall outcome is that wheat bran can be of help to some with constipation but for others with IBS it may make matters worse. It certainly can no longer be recommended as a cure-all for IBS.

Five years later *The Lancet* carried a report from a group of specialists at Addenbrooke's Hospital in Cambridge, led by Dr John Hunter, which told a rather different story. Their observation was that the avoidance of certain foods helped two-thirds of their

patients with IBS. Wheat was reported as the most common aggravating food and subsequent work has confirmed this initial observation. Wheat and its associated grains – oat, barley and rye – which all
contain the protein gluten, can cause either diarrhoea or constipation in a significant percentage of those with IBS. This effect seems
to take several days before it becomes apparent and may not be
noticed unless particular care is taken with the diet as a whole.

Further light was shed in the following year by Dr John Morley
and colleagues from Minneapolis in the United States. In a series of
experiments they showed that partially digested wheat contains a
substance that can actually slow the rate at which food passes
through the small bowel, where digestion takes place. This effect
was partially reversed by giving a drug that is an antidote to morphine and heroin. For some, wheat may act as 'a morphine-like drug'
– morphine's main side-effects are constipation and dopiness. So,
for some, wheat can irritate or even inflame the bowel and produce
diarrhoea. For others, it can actually aggravate constipation and for
others it is the cure. The first rule is that 'there are no rules'.

In other words, there is no obvious way of telling what adding
bran to the diet or increasing the dietary intake of wheat, oats, barley and rye will do to the sufferer of IBS. However, it is most unlikely to help diarrhoea, and there are safer and just as effective
types of fibre to take for constipation as we will see later in this
chapter.

## Tea

Is nothing sacred? This popular British beverage can also aggravate
constipation. On this occasion, it was not a group of English doctors,
but Scandinavians who revealed that, for approximately half of the
people in their study, replacing their daily intake of water with
several cups of tea per day slowed the rate at which food passed
from one end of the gut to the other. For the other half it made no difference. The effect that tea has on the gut is in broad terms the
opposite to that which coffee has.

## Dehydration

Lack of fluid is sometimes a cause of constipation. This is only likely
to happen if you spend any length of time in a hot climate, during
periods of very warm weather, in the elderly because they are
sometimes not aware of their needs, or if a fibre supplement is taken

without adequate fluid. If you do need to take a supplement of fibre, make sure that you drink one or two glasses of extra fluid per day.

## *Periods and hormones*

It is normal for the rate at which food moves through the gut to slow down in the week before the onset of menstruation. This may contribute to some women's abdominal bloating premenstrually. In those who experience this as part of their IBS, there can sometimes be a mild improvement if a supplement of Evening Primrose Oil is taken. Magnesium is also helpful (see below).

## —————————— Janet's story ——————————

Janet Duncan is a 44-year-old woman who works part time. When she came to the Women's Nutritional Advisory Service (WNAS) clinic she was suffering with Pre-Menstrual Syndrome (PMS), and had been suffering with abdominal bloating and pain for 15 years.

'My work was suffering as my symptoms were becoming worse and worse, so I felt I had to find a solution. My doctor had prescribed a water tablet, Burinex K, which I now gather has a side effect of causing a loss of the mineral magnesium. He also suggested that I take the contraceptive pill. As neither of these helped, in desperation I contacted the WNAS.

'I was told that the symptoms I was suffering with were very common and that they should respond to the programme within a matter of months. I was asked to cut out wheat, wheat-based products and processed foods from my diet, to exercise three or four times a week and to take the magnesium-rich multivitamin and mineral supplement, Optivite, daily. I followed the instructions religiously and found that I was considerably better within a few months, and completely over all the symptoms within six months.

'I tend to keep off wheat now, as I realize that it aggravates my symptoms. I am a great deal steadier mentally and physically.'

Our experience of seeing thousands of women at the WNAS, with PMS symptoms of mood swings, and physical symptoms such as abdominal bloating and breast tenderness, is that many of them have associated bowel problems. About 50 per cent complain of these. Constipation is more common than diarrhoea, and it seems that mental and physical symptoms of PMS are most likely to improve when the associated bowel problems are resolved. This may be due to possible effects on the function of hormones in some women with severe constipation.

Gut transit appears to be a little slower in women of child-bearing age when compared with those who are post-menopausal. This effect may be due to an effect of oestrogen on bowel function. Linseeds, which are a source of fibre but have oestrogen regulating effects, may be particularly useful in women whose constipation is perhaps affected by their hormonal state.

## *Magnesium*

This essential mineral was once used as a popular laxative in the form of Epsom Salts (which are magnesium sulphate). A relatively mild but consistent lack of this mineral has been reported as occurring in approximately 50 per cent of women with PMS. Supplements of magnesium, in the form of magnesium tablets or combined with multivitamins, are known to benefit PMS symptoms, and are likely to help overcome constipation as well.

Magnesium is a particularly interesting mineral when it comes to IBS and constipation because it is important for the chemical processes necessary for the relaxation of muscles. Deficiency can cause spasm of many muscles including the main muscles of the body such as in the arms, the legs, the back and the muscles in the walls of large blood vessels, which can then affect circulation. It is not known for certain what the effect of a relative lack of this mineral has on the gut. Our experience in many women with IBS and constipation – including a few with severe slow transit constipation – is that it is a simple, safe and effective laxative that combines well with a high fibre diet or with natural fibre supplements.

No one knows why magnesium levels are low in so many women with PMS and it would be interesting to know what the levels are like in those with constipation, especially if it is severe. But as yet, to our knowledge, no work has been done in this area. Magnesium's suitability as a laxative is confirmed by the fact that the main side-effect of magnesium tablets is diarrhoea.

## *Stress*

It probably won't be a surprise to you to read that stress affects the movement of food through the gut. One study has investigated the effect of stress on the contraction and relaxation of muscles in the small bowel, which is where digestion and absorption of nutrients take place. It was found that stress, in a variety of forms, reduced the number of effective contractions and increased the number of poorly co-ordinated spasm-like contractions in the small bowel of those with IBS. The effect on the colon was not recorded in this experiment, but it is likely to be very variable. To summarize, stress, which in this experiment included driving through London traffic, and playing a noisy arcade game, is likely to affect the way our gut works. Any stress can inhibit the normal regular contractions that occur spontaneously as part of an efficient digestive system, and increase the type of contractions that might aggravate bowel spasm and constipation.

## Pain

Quite understandably, pain of any type can disturb normal gut function. In some, it can probably switch off or diminish the desire to go to the toilet, and in others it may cause diarrhoea. Any painful pelvic condition, including ovarian cysts, endometriosis and period pains, can easily inhibit the urge to go to the toilet. Piles, or a tear in the margin of the anus or an anal fissure, are almost always associated with a powerful spasm of the muscles of the anal sphincter. This keeps the muscles of the lower end of the rectum and anus shut tight making it very difficult for a motion to pass. Sometimes these conditions can coexist with IBS, and they always need treating in their own right. For further advice on pain, see pages 46–51.

## Drugs

A number of drugs can cause constipation as a side-effect, including some which may be used to treat conditions associated with IBS. Common constipating preparations include anti-depressants and painkillers.

Anti-depressants are frequently accompanied by constipation, a dry mouth and sometimes blurred vision, especially at the start of therapy or if high doses are used. This effect is most noticeable with the older type of anti-depressants such as amitryptiline and desimipramine.

Strong painkillers – those that are derived from morphine – will invariably cause constipation. This means, for example, that any painkiller containing codeine or dihydrocodeine is likely to constipate.

As with diarrhoea if the constipation developed or worsened

shortly after you began taking a particular drug then ask your doctor about it. Usually stopping the drug for a week or two will result in a noticeable improvement.

## Exercise

It is becoming increasingly evident what a lazy nation we are. Lack of exercise is associated with being overweight, an increased risk of both heart disease and the likelihood of having a stroke, and is not good for the bowels. There is nothing like a good work-out to get the bowels functioning. If you haven't experienced it, and a sluggish colon is part of your problem, then it's time to give exercise a try (see page 69).

## Other foods

In addition to wheat and other grains, there is a wide variety of foods which can aggravate constipation and other symptoms of IBS. These are the same foods that by and large can aggravate diarrhoea. In short they can, in susceptible individuals, irritate the bowel. Whether this results in diarrhoea, constipation or a combination is dependent upon the person's own body chemistry and sensitivity.

Dr John Hunter and colleagues from Addenbrooke's Hospital in Cambridge have reported on their patients' experience of reaction to the following foods in terms of percentages.

| Food | % | Food | % | Food | % |
|------|-----|------|-----|------|-----|
| Wheat | 60 | Chocolate | 22 | Banana | 11 |
| Corn | 44 | Nuts | 22 | White fish | 10 |
| Milk | 44 | Potato | 20 | Shellfish | 10 |
| Cheese | 39 | Cabbage | 19 | Turnip | 10 |
| Oats | 34 | Beef | 16 | Tap water | 10 |
| Coffee | 33 | Rice | 15 | Turkey | 8 |
| Rye | 30 | Carrots | 15 | Marrow | 8 |
| Eggs | 26 | Pork | 14 | Smoked fish | 7 |
| Tea | 25 | Chicken | 13 | Pear | 7 |
| Citrus | 24 | Apple | 12 | Melon | 5 |
| Yoghurt | 24 | Yeast | 12 | Avocado | 5 |
| Barley | 24 | Lamb | 11 | Honey | 2 |
| Onion | 22 | | | | |

Almost every food tried seemed to cause problems for some patients, but this should be interpreted with caution. As a rule, percentage figures of ten per cent or below are not necessarily that meaningful. The only way to be sure that a particular food causes upset is if it does so repeatedly or if the presence of a true allergy is confirmed by a blood test. This was not the case at this stage of Dr Hunter's assessment but the data do provide a useful guide to the likely percentage of IBS sufferers who may have a problem with these foods.

Because diet can play such an important part in the alleviation of IBS symptoms, it is often advisable for those with troublesome IBS to follow a formal dietary experiment. You can learn to determine which foods are causing you problems by following the ten-week diet which begins on page 104. You will also need to take into account any of your own particular observations about your bowels and diet. For example, if you know that mangoes or tomatoes upset you then leave them out. Trust your own judgement. Remember it's your body, and you will know it better than anyone else.

# Diarrhoea and IBS

## Andrea's story

Andrea had been suffering with IBS for a year and a half, following a bout of food poisoning.

'I was left with awful diarrhoea after an episode of food poisoning. The doctor said it would pass, but it didn't. I used to get very bloated, with lots of wind and pain, and would have diarrhoea about four times each day, which left me utterly drained and exhausted. The only medication I took was codeine phosphate, which helped to ease the pain a little.

'Through the WNAS I discovered that my diet was responsible for my symptoms. When I cut out wheat, especially bran flakes and granary bread, my symptoms disappeared. I noticed that spicy and sugary foods, as well as coffee, can bring on the symptoms. In fact I got caught out after having a curry – never again!

'I don't eat any muesli or wholemeal bread now as it makes me feel bloated, windy and awful. I eat lots of fruit and vegetables so that I don't get constipated, and as long as I stick to my diet, I feel fine.'

---

In addition to the basic dietary and other recommendations, there are some points that need a special mention for those for whom diarrhoea is the main symptom.

Diarrhoea means having frequent or loose stools. 'Frequent' is if you have more than three stools per day, and 'loose' means anything that is not formed, from the consistency of soft putty to watery. Diarrhoea mainly occurs because food has moved too quickly through the gut and there has not been time for the water in the bowel to be absorbed.

In IBS, diarrhoea certainly can be due to an intolerance or reaction to certain foods and these are listed below.

**Milk** can cause bowel problems, and in particular diarrhoea, in one of two ways. Some people, especially children and infants, may react to the protein in milk and this can cause abdominal pain (or colic in an infant), and sometimes diarrhoea. Other signs of allergy that may be present are eczema, asthma or rhinitis.

Sometimes there can be a problem with milk sugar (lactose). If this is not able to be digested then the sugar passes into the small bowel and colon where it acts as a potent laxative. Often the severely affected sufferer is troubled with diarrhoea within an hour of consuming milk or soft cheese, although hard cheese or small amounts of milk may be tolerated. This type of food intolerance is quite common in those of Eastern European, Middle Eastern or Asian origin and in others it can temporarily follow an episode of acute gastroenteritis. Drinking skimmed or semi-skimmed milk makes no difference to either cow's milk protein or lactose intolerance as it is only the fat content that is reduced in these milks and not the protein or sugar content.

## Ruth's story

Ruth was an anxious 53-year-old who had started to experience diarrhoea and weight loss after a stomach operation. Earlier in the year she had noticed indigestion after meals and a subsequent investigation showed some inflammation of the lower end of the oesophagus (gullet). This had the potential to become cancerous and meant that she then needed an operation to remove it. The operation had gone smoothly enough but afterwards her weight fell from 70 kg (11 stone) to 50 kg (8 stone) and she noticed that quite severe diarrhoea would follow when eating certain meals.

The pattern of her symptoms strongly suggested that she now had trouble with milk products. For example, on several occasions she had tried drinking a glass of milk to help put her weight back on, and this had resulted in diarrhoea and wind about 30 minutes later. This was almost certainly due to a difficulty in the digestion of milk sugar (lactose).

Ruth was advised to eat a low dairy diet and avoid foods with added milk or that contained lactose. Because this would mean a significant fall in her intake of calcium, she was also advised to take a calcium supplement providing between 500 and 1000 mg per day. This is essential advice for children and middle-aged or elderly women on a low dairy or dairy-free diet. Poor dietary intake of calcium can, after many years, lead to osteoporosis – thinning of the bones and fractures.

Some people with true lactose intolerance may be able to tolerate lactose-free milk, which is available in some supermarkets; hard cheeses, as they have relatively small amounts of lactose; and be helped by adding Lactaid (available from chemists and health food shops) to ordinary milk. A few drops of this preparation helps break down lactose into its two component sugars, glucose and galactose, which are easily absorbed without causing diarrhoea.

**Wheat and other grains**  It now seems that wheat – together with the other gluten-containing grains, oats, barley and rye – is one of the most common foods which aggravates the symptoms of IBS. In addition, sensitivity to these cereals has also been recorded as a cause of diarrhoea especially in women. This is by no means accepted as conventional medical wisdom, even though a group of ten such patients were described as long ago as 1980 by one leading group of gastroenterologists from Birmingham in the UK. It would seem that some very sensitive individuals do react to wheat which can cause some minor but definite damage to the lining of the gut and result in diarrhoea. This situation is similar to, but not the same as, coeliac disease in which the degree of gluten sensitivity is even more severe. Interestingly, it has been shown recently that rice actually inhibits the secretion of watery fluids into the gut and may be helpful in the recovery from diarrhoea. This has long been used in Third World countries and has been adopted in the United Kingdom to help the rate of recovery in children with acute infectious diarrhoea.

In the diet section rice is normally allowed and may specifically help some patients with diarrhoea.

**Eating a large meal**  that distends the stomach causes a reflex contraction of the muscles of the colon. This is known as the gastro-colic reflex, and explains why some of us most often feel the need to open our bowels within an hour of our main meal of the day. It isn't the meal we have just eaten coming through already but probably the day before's moving on. Some are unduly sensitive in this way.

**Fatty foods – too much and too little**  If the digestion is poor, too much fatty food can lead to diarrhoea. This is most evident in those with known digestive problems, and in the elderly, especially if there is weight loss. The fat that is not digested in the small bowel can be broken down into irritating acids by bacteria in the large bowel. Some may experience diarrhoea a few hours after eating a large or rich meal.

Conversely, fat in more modest quantities actually slows down the rate at which the stomach empties and food moves along the small bowel. It takes time to digest fat in a meal and so the gut is sensitive to its presence. Certain fats seem particularly prone to this. Oleic acid, which is found in olive oil, almonds, hazel nuts, Brazil nuts and avocado pears, slows down the rate at which food moves through the small bowel. It is thought that too low a fat intake may explain why low-fat diets in children can prolong toddler diarrhoea. Furthermore, consumption of low-fat cow's milk in children is strongly associated with an increase in acute gastroenteritis infections.

So the answer seems to be not too much nor too little. It would be prudent to limit your fat intake if you have diarrhoea and are overweight and to make sure that you have enough if you are underweight. If you are underweight, you should also try to eat nutritious fat-containing foods at each meal, and snacks in between. Examples of these are nuts, seeds, oily fish, lean meat, dairy products, and salad dressings made with olive oil.

**Coffee**, an extremely popular beverage, is also an excellent bowel stimulant. Ordinary and even decaffeinated coffee have effects on the gut. One of these actions is to stimulate a wave of contraction along the bowel, and many of us use a cup of coffee as a way of helping us to go to the toilet. However, for some it can actually be a cause of diarrhoea, so if you have diarrhoea and you drink coffee you should cut down your intake or stop it completely. This includes decaffeinated coffee as well as it too can affect the gut.

**Hot drinks** can also stimulate a wave of contraction through the bowel. So again it may be necessary to limit the number of such drinks that you have.

**Fruit** Many of us know that too much fruit can be a cause of diarrhoea. This may be because it is difficult for the upper bowel to absorb large amounts of fruit sugar – fructose – completely. Studies have examined the effect of fructose, or honey, a rich natural source of fructose, on the bowel. In one experiment doses of either 50 g (1¾ oz) or 100 g (3½ oz) of honey resulted in 10 per cent of the sugar content not being absorbed. For many subjects mild abdominal bloating, increase in wind and possibly subsequent diarrhoea would follow. In children, excessive consumption of fruit juices are a known cause of toddler diarrhoea and carbohydrates, other than fructose, are also thought to be factors. The solution to this problem is simply to have small amounts, say one or two pieces of fruit at a time, and allow two or three hours to elapse before having more.

**Artificial sweeteners** like sorbitol, which is used in some sugar-free chewing gums and sweets, especially mints, can cause diarrhoea, if consumed excessively. Sorbitol is an 'artificial sugar' which tastes sweet but cannot be digested. It therefore passes through the small bowel intact, moving on to the large bowel where it can attract water in the same way that some mineral laxatives do. So eating too many low-calorie mints can be a cause of diarrhoea.

**Spicy foods** can act as potential laxatives by stimulating the bowel. Many people would include a number of Indian spices in this category but this is not always the case. One study has shown that both red chilli and cayenne pepper actually slow the rate at which food moves along the small bowel, possibly allowing more time for digestion. But others may report the opposite effect upon their colon, so trust your own observations and judgements. What suits one may not suit another.

**Smoking cigarettes** is known to increase the contraction of the colon muscles in those with IBS. If you smoke, or have been a smoker, you will know that a few puffs can cause a need to open the bowels. For many, a cup of coffee and a cigarette is their way of instigating going to the toilet. Smoking also increases the level of acid in the stomach and causes acid to wash back into the oesophagus. It is a prime cause of indigestion and peptic ulcers.

**Alcohol** can also sometimes cause diarrhoea, but usually this is only likely to happen in those who drink very heavily. One unit of alcohol equals one glass of wine or half a pint of ordinary strength beer. The safe limit for men is three units per day and for women it is two. Intakes higher than this are associated with a number of health problems, from liver disease to an increased risk of cancer, and alcohol knocks most nutrients sideways.

Sometimes certain alcoholic beverages can aggravate IBS because of a sensitivity to yeast. This is possible with beer, especially yeasty tasting real ales. Men are more likely to be victims and this is not a common problem.

### _____ Theresa's story _____

Theresa was a middle-aged lady from Ireland who had had her share of troubles over the years. On and off for two decades she had been depressed and had been on anti-depressant drugs for most of this time. Her depression had often been related to her drinking, which had been excessive in the past but had now settled down to about three double whiskies a day. For the last year she noticed that her abdomen was becoming distended, that her stools were looser and that she needed to go to the toilet up to six times each day. The diarrhoea was controlled in part by drugs and she had noticed a slight benefit if she avoided dairy products. A specialist had investigated her thoroughly and found no serious problem. It had been concluded that she had IBS with a possible intolerance of lactose.

When Theresa attended the clinic, the best approach seemed to be to advise her to avoid a variety of other foods for two weeks, since a number of food intolerances might be causing her diarrhoea, but this was without benefit. Because of the combination of long-standing depression and more recent diarrhoea it seemed prudent to check her level of vitamin B, especially vitamin B3 as a lack of this can cause both depression and diarrhoea and is more likely in those who regularly drink alcohol.

Her test result was low and she was recommended to take strong supplements of vitamin B complex and extra vitamin B3, and to reduce her alcohol consumption. Within three weeks the diarrhoea had settled greatly and she felt much better in herself. The improvement was sustained over two years. She seemed able to tolerate milk products without any problems but some depression remained. Her abnormally low vitamin B3 level returned to normal.

It seems that Theresa's lack of vitamin B3 was to a large degree due to her alcohol consumption of six or more units a day. It was surprising that this had occurred because she had an excellent diet, and had not developed the typical red scaly rash on her face and hands that is characteristic of a vitamin B3 deficiency. Mild deficiencies of B vitamins do occur at a level that produces symptoms without any other features.

Though deficiency of vitamin B3 is rare, it is worth bearing in mind if diarrhoea is associated with depression, or you regularly consume alcohol.

**Surgery** may upset the gut. Many operations on the stomach or bowel can leave the owner with a tendency to diarrhoea. This is particularly true if part of the stomach or small bowel is removed or if the nerves to the stomach have been cut. The need for many of these operations has fallen dramatically over the last decade because of improvements in drug therapy. Specialist advice and treatment are required from a doctor in these situations.

Bowel disturbance can occasionally follow surgery for gall stones but this usually settles with time.

**Drugs and vitamins**    can occasionally cause diarrhoea as a side-effect – antibiotics are common and well-known examples. This can be due to their killing off friendly bacteria in the colon, which can allow unfriendly bacteria or yeasts to proliferate. These in turn can produce irritant substances which overstimulate the colon producing diarrhoea. This is more likely if several antibiotics are taken either together or one after another. The diarrhoea usually lasts for a few days only, but can sometimes continue for several weeks and be associated with weight loss and an inability to digest fatty foods. Some erythromycins can cause diarrhoea because they help to stimulate the muscles of the bowel. This antibiotic is quite often used in children and in the treatment of acne.

Many other drugs can also cause diarrhoea including those used to treat arthritis and other painful conditions, to lower raised cholesterol levels, and to treat high blood pressure, as well as other conditions. The obvious clue is if the diarrhoea starts shortly after the drug is begun. Stopping the drug should result in improvement within a few days, though occasionally this may take longer. The recovery from antibiotic-induced diarrhoea is apparently quicker if supplements of vitamin B complex are also taken.

Nutritional supplements, particularly large doses of vitamin C and magnesium, can cause diarrhoea. Some people can be troubled by yeast tablets, iron or multivitamins with iron. Again, the clue is if the diarrhoea starts shortly after the supplements are taken. The effect of iron and magnesium can, however, be delayed for several weeks or months.

## Barbara's story

Barbara came to the WNAS clinic at the suggestion of her General Practitioner because of her recurrent oral thrush and IBS. For three years she had experienced a sore mouth with a white deposit on the tongue, swabs from which had shown a growth of *Candida albicans*. She had also had several episodes of vaginal thrush which required treatment. Over this time she had experienced bouts of diarrhoea up to five times a day and these seemed to be related to eating certain foods but the pattern was not clear to her. From her own interpretation, she strongly suspected that she was sensitive to yeast.

However she did not seem to have any active yeast infection, and tests for anaemia, iron and zinc deficiency and diabetes were all normal, so there did not appear to be any nutritional problems that predisposed her to thrush infections. Adhering strictly to a diet avoiding yeast and yeast-derived foods completely controlled her symptoms. Addition of these foods back into her diet revealed that she was exquisitely sensitive: bread and any type of alcohol-based drink, including low-alcohol lager, caused abdominal bloating and diarrhoea by the next day. Pickled onions caused mouth burning, probably because of their vinegar content, but pasta and soda bread were fine.

An additional benefit was that if she was careful with her diet for the whole month then her periods were less heavy and painful. Some of the chemicals released from the gut as part of true food intolerance reactions are the same as those involved in period pains. It is possible that what irritates the bowel may irritate the uterus.

**Monthly periods** may also be associated with diarrhoea. This may be due to the release of chemicals that stimulate the bowel to contract as well as the uterus.

These factors should be taken into account if you have diarrhoea as one of your main symptoms. You will need to follow the main diet for IBS on page 104 and need to incorporate some of the above factors. You will also find some practical tips for overcoming diarrhoea on pages 86–87.

# Pain and IBS

## Sonya's story

Sonya Martin is a 33-year-old administrator who lives in Sussex. She is married and has two children. She has had severe problems with her periods since her teens and later developed IBS.

'During my first pregnancy I was anaemic and suffered with severe constipation and piles. In my second pregnancy, I had prolapsed piles and I remember thinking that I wouldn't wish that condition on my worst enemy. I would hold my baby in my arms, and crawl along the floor, because I couldn't walk.

'I used to suffer with severe abdominal pains following this. One night I had an attack of the most terrible abdominal pain, so bad that I wanted to die. The doctor was called, and by the time he arrived I was hyperventilating. An ambulance was called, and I was taken to casualty, writhing and groaning in pain. The examining doctor was surprised by the amount of pain I was in, and was unable to make a diagnosis. I was kept in overnight for observation and given painkillers. The following morning, I was sent home with a diagnosis of colic of the bowel, and no follow-up treatment whatsoever.

'I have now been attending the WNAS clinic for five months. I followed a diet, exercise and supplement programme that was designed for me, and within only the first month I noticed a spectacular difference. I now have no bowel problems at all, and no period problems either. I continue to avoid wheat-based products, which seem to cause my problems, and to take my supplements and exercise. I can honestly say that I feel better than I have felt for years, and I am immensely grateful. I do wish that the doctors I saw over the years had been armed with adequate knowledge about diet, which would have saved me a lot of pain and trauma.'

## Jane's story

Jane Donn is a 43-year-old woman from Glasgow. She works as a customer service officer in a bank and has two children. She had been suffering with IBS for three years and had four episodes of hospitalization as a result of her symptoms. She contacted the WNAS in September 1993.

'I suffered with severe abdominal pain, bloating and wind, and I regularly used to vomit after meals, especially if I ate after 5 pm. I was always constipated and was only able to go to the toilet once or twice a week. My symptoms used to ruin my life. The last two years our summer holidays have been spoiled as I have spent at least a week in bed each time. I have lost count of the number of social occasions I have had to cancel. All of this was bad for me, but equally bad for my husband and my daughters who have had to live with it.

'My doctor diagnosed IBS, and prescribed Regulan, lactulose and Colofac. He suggested that I eat plenty of bran, wholemeal bread and fruit, and rest in bed when the attacks were bad. Due to the extreme pain, I was admitted to hospital in August, September and December of 1990, and again for three weeks in May 1993. I remember having tubes coming out of every orifice, and being given strong painkillers, which made me even more sick. The whole thing was such a nightmare as I felt so out of control.

'Then I read a newspaper article about the research the WNAS had been doing and contacted them. Within one week of starting my programme I felt significantly better – I had much more energy and no bowel symptoms. I now know that the bran and the wholemeal bread were not tolerated by my gut.

'I don't eat any wheat products now and avoid tea and coffee. I am so much better that I have no desire to try to reintroduce them at the moment. I no longer vomit after meals, and I can regularly go out for meals in the evening with no ill effect. I even went to a dinner dance until 1 am recently, which is something I would never have been able to do before. I don't take any medication now, just Linusit Gold with my cereals, and this keeps the constipation at bay. As well as overcoming the IBS, my periods have regulated, and I no longer have insomnia. I sleep like a baby each night, it's bliss.'

---

Pain, usually somewhere in the abdomen, is a common but not universal symptom of IBS. Any pain is nature's way of telling us that something is wrong, and the pain in IBS can be anything from a mild ache to – less usually – a severe cramp-like pain. It can be felt almost anywhere in the abdomen, from underneath the ribs to low down just above the pubic bone, and it can be on either side of the abdomen. Low back pain can also occur as part of IBS.

There have been several attempts by doctors to determine the cause of the pain in IBS. These experiments have involved volunteers swallowing a fine tube which passes through the small intestine. At set points a balloon on the end of this tube is inflated so that it presses on the walls of the intestine and there is a rise in pressure inside both the balloon and the gut. Some experiments have involved a balloon being passed into the colon from the back passage and similarly being inflated. What the brave volunteer always notices is pain.

Often a point somewhere in the small bowel can be found where inflation of the balloon exactly reproduces the pain that that person experiences as part of his or her IBS. This has led many researchers to conclude that much of the pain of IBS is due to a rise in pressure in the bowel, almost certainly as a result of poorly co-ordinated contractions of the muscles in the wall of the bowel. Furthermore, as far as the pain goes the small bowel is just as likely to be at fault as the colon or large bowel. The evidence from this type of experiment is very convincing. Whatever else is going on, the pain at least is likely to be due in part or in whole to physical factors, and it is not 'all in the mind' as may previously have been considered.

One group of doctors investigated a group of ten women with IBS, whose main symptoms were abdominal pain and bloating. The rate at which their waste material moved through the first part of the colon, the caecum, was delayed. Once again it seemed that there was not always a satisfactory wave of effective contraction of the muscles of the gut in this region. It is surprising that these doctors used a radioactive form of wheat bran to look at the function of the gut – food now known to be more likely to aggravate rather than help the symptoms of IBS. Spasm in this region of the bowel may result in pain concentrated in the lower right-hand part of the abdomen, which could also be sensitive when pressed.

Spasm can occur as well in the lower end of the colon which may be felt as pain in the lower left-hand part of the abdomen. This area may also be tender to the touch, and in thin people it may be possible to feel part of the bowel in this region. Spasm in this area of the colon seems often to be associated with constipation and the passing of a pellety stool. Pain could also be due to other related changes in the bowel. A build-up of wind in the colon will cause a rise in pressure which could easily be felt as pain or discomfort. Pain of this sort may be relieved by the passage of wind.

In those with true food intolerance there can be a release from the wall of the bowel of chemicals that stimulate inflammation. These chemicals are the same as those that are produced in arthritis and other situations where the tissues are irritated and trying to heal. They could certainly cause or aggravate pain.

Another possible cause of pain in IBS is an increase in the tension of the muscles in the floor of the pelvis. These are the muscles that we use to help control our passing of water and opening our bowels. They need to relax when we wish to perform these functions, and if they do not then pain on going to the toilet is the likely result. This pain can be felt low down in the abdomen, in the small of the back, or in the region of the front or back passage.

In the main then, it seems that most of the pain in IBS is due to a build-up of pressure which is often due to irregular and poorly co-ordinated contraction of the muscles of the gut. For some with IBS, pain is most evident when there is also a need to open the bowels. Pain is then typically felt in the lower part of the abdomen, and is probably related to the contraction of the muscles in the lower part of the bowel. The passage of waste material from the end of the colon into the rectum results in the feeling of wanting to open the bowels. It also results in a nerve reflex that relaxes the muscles at the lower end of the rectum and the anus. This is a powerful reflex and it can help overcome the spasm that some IBS sufferers experience in this region. This is an opportunity for the constipated IBS sufferer to open their bowels relatively easily, and should not be ignored. Failure to comply with this message is likely to cause increasing pressure and indeed pain in the lower part of the bowel without any useful result. Mother nature's advice is to accept the invitation and go with the flow!

So much for the nitty gritty of pain from the bowels, but there is another important aspect too. Pain is a complicated sensation. As well as being due to pressure or damage to a tissue, it is also greatly influenced by a person's state of mind. There are parts of the brain which alter our perception of pain, and this in turn is influenced by a person's mental state. In general, anything that increases the person's degree of introversion such as personal worries, being told by their doctor that their pain is 'just imaginary', or even thinking that there is nothing that they can do about their problems, is likely to increase the level of pain perceived. Conversely, activities that distract the individual's attention away from their worries and pain are likely to help. Pleasurable activities can help to displace the feeling of pain.

Dr Chambers and Dr Bland from London noticed that many of those attending hospital with IBS were also experiencing the symptoms of hyperventilation or overbreathing. In hyperventilating there is a subtle – though sometimes obvious – alteration in the rate and pattern of breathing. This causes slight chemical changes in the body and can be associated with an increased level of anxiety, feelings of breathlessness, palpitations and increased sensitivity to pain. If this description fits you to some degree then controlled breathing exercises can help you to limit these problems. Often these symptoms occur as part of a panic attack or a painful experience such as an episode of bowel spasm.

Understanding the underlying causes of the pain in IBS should help you, possibly with the help of your doctor, to come up with approaches that are effective in reducing it.

## *Ways to reduce the pain of IBS*

- Tackle the factors that cause or aggravate constipation. See Chapter 5. This alone may be enough for many with IBS.
- Avoid any foods that you know or strongly suspect aggravate any of your IBS symptoms including diarrhoea and wind.
- Avoid painkillers that contain codeine or related compounds. Their main side-effect is constipation, which is likely to make things worse in the long run. Paracetamol is more likely to be suitable but should only be taken as a short-term measure.
- Ask your doctor to prescribe a medicine with anti-spasm properties. One, based on peppermint (Colpermin), can be moderately helpful.
- Try taking a regular daily supplement of magnesium. This is essential if you are constipated despite making changes to your diet. Magnesium in the form of amino acid chelate, gluconate or oxide seems particularly appropriate. A reasonable dose is 200 mg two or three times a day. The only likely side-effect of taking too much is diarrhoea.
- Never ignore the urge to open your bowels! If you hear the call, go, or be prepared to suffer the consequences.
- Relax. Even if you are in pain, try to relax. Sit down, lie down or go to sleep if you can. Yoga, self-hypnosis, or listening to some of your favourite music can all help. Find out what works for you.
- Have a hot bath. This is one of the best ways to relax and it also helps to ease tension in the muscles of both the gut and the pelvis.
- Try using a hot-water bottle or a heat pad, which you can carry around with you and even take to work. Applying heat to a painful and troubled abdomen can help to soothe the pain.

- Have a massage. Gentle massage of the lower back can help ease the pain for some. Sometimes a very light massage of the abdomen can be helpful too. This should always be in a clockwise motion, the direction of flow through the colon.
- Treat any painful condition affecting the anus. This may mean seeing your doctor to get treatment for your piles. Glycerine suppositories are a simple way of helping to overcome constipation due to painful anal conditions.
- Try a cup of Rooibosch tea made from the South African red bush. One variety of this caffeine-free low tannin 'tea', called Eleven O'clock, has been shown to have a relaxing effect on the gut muscle and has been used to treat colic in babies.

It is worth mentioning that if the pain is long-standing and is associated with feelings of depression or anxiety, you should see your doctor. Sometimes a small dose of an anti-depressant drug can have useful painkilling properties, but it has to be a small dose because large doses can cause constipation. Use of this type of drug should not stop you and your doctor from looking at the way that dietary and other factors may be influencing your IBS.

As with the other treatment recommendations, it is often necessary to combine a number of these approaches before you find those that are helpful to you. Be patient. It can take several weeks before some of these treatments work.

Remember also that if your pain is severe, or if it changes, then you should check with your doctor if you have not done so already.

# Wind and bloating

Abdominal bloating is one of the most common symptoms of IBS and is often, though not always, accompanied by excessive wind. By wind we mean flatus, or gas passed through the back passage. Burping, or to give it its medical term, eructation, can occur as part of IBS and is usually due to the swallowing of air.

To the relief of many sufferers, who in the past have been accused of bad posture, a recent study has confirmed that much of the bloating of the abdomen that takes place in IBS is due to a build-up of gas in the bowel. This comes from the breakdown of both food residues in the colon and also from the residue of mucus or digestive slime and juices that our own intestines produce. Consequently bloating can still persist even if you have not eaten anything for a day or two.

This chapter is about the factors that can contribute to this production of gas in the bowel.

## Susan's story

Susan Stevens is a 33-year-old housewife from London, who has two children. When she came to the WNAS clinic, she had been suffering with severe abdominal bloating and wind for over six months.

'I used to bloat up and get terrible wind for no apparent reason. I would swell so much that I could not fit into my clothes, which I found very annoying. It always used to happen when I was about to go out, and I would be left feeling unsightly with nothing to wear. I went to see my doctor, who prescribed "water" tablets, spironolactone, for the bloating. I took these, but didn't find that they helped much, and I still had the painful wind.

'I started my course with the WNAS in the spring of 1993. I was put on a basic diet to start with and noticed a significant improvement within the first month. I discovered that sweet things like puddings, sweets, biscuits, cakes and rye products gave me wind. I use LoSalt, instead of salt, when I really fancy a salty flavour.

'I spend time each week exercising and relaxing and now feel fitter generally and not so tensed up with people and life. I have been able to cheat occasionally without rocking the boat. Occasionally, when I am entertaining, I do eat foods that I know upset me, and it takes me a few days to get the feeling of well-being afterwards. As a result of this treatment, I have learned how to tune in to my body, and seem to know when I can cross the line and when I can't. I have my figure back, I no longer have the embarrassment of the wind, and my self-esteem has improved dramatically.'

# Wind in the bowels

First, here's a bit of science on the subject of wind production, which has only been taken seriously in the last decade. A variety of gases are produced by the billions of mainly friendly bacteria that inhabit the large colon. They are found only in very small amounts in the small bowel where the majority of digestion and absorption of nutrients takes place. They first appear in any quantity in the cae-cum, which is the first part of the large bowel and is found on the right side of your abdomen, in the lower part at the point where your appendix is (if you have still got it).

Here, the bacteria sit waiting to see what will turn up in the form of leftovers from the meal that you have eaten several hours before. No matter how efficient your digestion is, there is always something left over. This constitutes about five to fifteen per cent of our intake of fat, protein and carbohydrate and all of the fibre. A number of in-teresting, and at times peculiar, things happen when this supply of nutrients reaches the bacteria in the colon. There are, in fact, more bacteria in the colon than there are cells in the body, and this bacterial Mafia has a way of dealing with the supply of leftover food that is very different to the body's metabolism.

The most noticeable difference is that many of these bacteria pro-duce gases that our own cells are, for the most part, incapable of producing. They include hydrogen, methane, and carbon dioxide, all of which have no smell. In some people and under certain circum-stances bad-eggs gas, hydrogen sulphide, is produced – an event with which some of us are doubtlessly familiar. Curiously there is a difference between people living in the West compared with those from the East. We all produce hydrogen, but only a proportion of those in the West produce methane, and many others produce hydrogen sulphide or bad-eggs gas instead. This is influenced by our diets in the West – it is not just the industrial factories that are re-sponsible for some of our more noxious emissions.

In addition to the gases, there are a number of simple fats that are produced which can be absorbed into the body and can provide some two to five per cent of our daily energy needs. So we do get something useful back too. Also, a large amount of water and a small amount of some minerals are slowly absorbed in the colon.

So there is quite a lot of activity in the normal colon, and in many ways it is comparable to the rumen of cattle such as sheep and cows. They have several stomachs which contain bacteria whose main function is to assist in the breakdown of the tough fibre-rich grasses and plants that they eat. Their digestions enlist the help of similar friendly bacteria except that they are in the first part of their intestines and not at the end as in ours. Everyone has some wind but the amount and type can vary greatly.

# What influences the production of wind?

We don't wish to dwell on science, but this is a very complicated subject. Understanding the factors that influence the activity of the bacteria in the colon may be of importance not only in IBS, but also in cancer of the colon, certain types of arthritis and even cholesterol metabolism. What goes on in the bowel can influence many aspects of body health. The amount and the type of wind that any one individual produces is influenced by:

- The type of food eaten, especially fibre rich foods.
- How well the food is digested in the small bowel.
- How quickly food and food residues pass through the small bowel to reach the colon.
- The type of bacteria present in the colon. This is also influenced by the type of diet you eat, presence or absence of illness, use of antibiotics and even the type of bacteria in the colons of those with whom you live.

The factors that influence wind production are highly variable from person to person. This has been observed in just about every study that has taken a look at this problem. What gives wind to one person will often have no effect on others. And even the susceptible person may well find that under certain circumstances he or she is able to tolerate foods that have previously been a source of discomfort or embarrassment. Again, it appears to be a combination of factors rather than any single one that is often relevant.

Excessive production of wind is more likely to occur if:

- You eat foods to which you are intolerant – in theory this could be any food depending upon your individual sensitivities.
- You eat foods that contain sugars that you cannot easily digest. For example, those who cannot digest lactose develop diarrhoea and wind if they drink milk. The undigested milk sugar is rapidly fermented by the bacteria in the large bowel to produce a lot of gas and some acids which stimulate and irritate the bowel. The same can happen on rare occasions in some susceptible individuals with the following sugars and carbohydrates: ordinary table sugar – sucrose (found in most sweets and sweetened foods); fruit sugar or fructose (found in most fruits and vegetables); the artificial sweetener Sorbitol (found in cool-tasting mints and some sugar-free sweets) taken in excess.
- You eat foods that are known to be hard to digest, especially if they are not well cooked or eaten in large amounts. This is potentially a long list and includes for many: wheat especially wheat bran and wholewheat products; coarse oats, barley and rye; sweet corn especially if whole and not chewed well; brown rice; potatoes (sometimes); beans (not green), lentils and sometimes peas; vegetables of the *Brassica* family – cabbage, cauliflower, broccoli and Brussels sprouts; Jerusalem artichokes; shells of prawns and other crustacea; mushrooms (sometimes); onions, leeks, garlic and asparagus.
- You have a rapid rate of small bowel gut transit. This is more likely in men than in women and as already mentioned can be speeded up by drinking a lot of coffee and possibly aggravated by eating a very large meal. A low fat high carbohydrate, high fibre diet might make this worse too. The combination of rapid passage through the small bowel of a meal that was hard to digest will mean that the bacteria of the colon are going to get their full share.
- You have a poor digestion. Weight loss and or abdominal pain after eating should prompt you to see your doctor without delay.
- You make excessive use of laxatives.
- You take certain drugs. Some recently introduced drugs inhibit the digestion of sugar and are used in the treatment of diabetes. An all too predictable side-effect is abdominal wind and bloating.
- You eat large amounts of caramel, burnt sugar and modified starch and have a sensitive digestion. These have all been chemically altered by heat or the cooking process which makes them

hard for some people to digest. Caramel is widely used as a colouring and flavouring agent (read all labels), and there are significant amounts in most beers.

So, if you want to try to reduce the amount of wind that you produce you should:

1  Eat slowly and chew your food well.
2  Avoid foods that you know upset you.
3  Make sure that your vegetables are not undercooked.
4  If you eat beans soak them overnight, shake them to remove the husks and cook them thoroughly. Many, including red kidney beans, need to be cooked for at least ten minutes on a rolling boil and then simmered for an hour before they are ready to eat. This reduces the potential wind-producing culprits – two tough carbohydrates called stacchyose and raffinose. Black-eyed beans and red kidney beans are more likely to cause wind than other varieties. Fresh or frozen peas are usually well tolerated.
5  Avoid eating very large meals. It may be easier on your digestion to eat little and often and to give yourself some stress-free time afterwards to help it digest.
6  Avoid foods rich in sulphur and sulphites. These chemicals encourage the conversion of hydrogen in the colon to hydrogen sulphide, bad-eggs gas.
   The main dietary sources of these chemicals are
- Bread.
- Foods preserved with sulphur dioxide e.g. dried fruits, fruit squash drinks and anything else containing a sulphite or meta-bisulphite compound (you'll need to read the label).
- Wines, beers and cider which again often contain sulphite as a preservative (never mentioned on the label due to the absence of any EEC regulation for alcoholic beverages).
- Sulphur-rich foods including eggs and all members of the onion family.

Small amounts of these are usually tolerated until the excess reaches the colonic bacteria.

Listed below are some common foods, with their sulphur dioxide content in parts per million, plus the chemical name of E numbers containing sulphur.

| | | | |
|---|---|---|---|
| Pizza dough | 10-20 | Molasses | 125 |
| Instant tea | 5-6 | Beer | 10 |
| Wine vinegar | 75 | Wine | 150 |
| Fresh shrimp | 4-36 | E220 | Sulphur Dioxide |
| Grapes | 15 | E221 | Sodium Sulphite |
| Dried fruits (apples, raisins) | 275 | E222 | Sodium Hydrogen |
| Grape juice | 85 | | Sulphite |
| Lemon juice | 800 | E223 | Sodium Metabisulphite |
| Canned vegetables | 5-30 | E224 | Potassium Metabisulphite |
| Instant potatoes | 35-90 | E226 | Calcium Sulphite |
| Corn syrup | 30 | E227 | Calcium Hydrogen |
| Fruit toppings | 60 | | Sulphite |

7  Avoid caramel, burnt sugar and foods containing them.

8  Avoid smoking heavily during or after a large meal. This can inhibit digestive function and for some could result in increased wind production.

9  Try taking charcoal biscuits. This old-fashioned remedy might help if you are lucky.

10  Try taking live yoghurt. This is rich in certain semi-friendly bacteria. Better than the worst that might live in your bowel but not always the best. It is inadvisable for those who have had surgery on the gut, especially if part of the small bowel has been removed, to eat large amounts of this or take preparations containing lactobacillus bacteria. They can make the gut contents too acidic.

11  Swallow your pride and see your doctor. Persistent, excessive and offensive wind may be the first sign of a digestive problem for which a change in diet may not be enough.

12  Be patient. Some of these changes to your diet could take several weeks to have an effect. Up to six weeks is a reasonable time span.

# 9

# Medical treatments for IBS

Although this book is not primarily about drug treatments, you need to know about them. As you will see there are many preparations that tackle IBS in different ways. There isn't *one* good treatment for IBS but there are several different treatments and some of these do have some true value. Most of them are chosen by doctors on the basis of the type of symptoms that the patient has. The types of treatment are:

- Laxatives
- Anti-diarrhoea drugs
- Anti-wind drugs
- Anti-spasm drugs
- Drugs that help stimulate the muscles of the gut.

## *Laxatives*

There are three main types of laxative, which can be classified as bulk laxatives, stimulant laxatives and stool softeners.

### Bulk laxatives

These work by increasing the size of the stool and making it easier to pass. They retain a certain amount of water and give bulk to the stool. This in turn helps to stimulate the bowel muscles into a normal level of activity. These preparations are useful for those with constipation who either pass stools infrequently, pass very hard stools or thin misshapen stools, or who have to strain to go to the toilet. Bulk laxatives include:

### *Bran*

This is the outer indigestible part of the wheat husk. It is what is normally thrown away when wheat or other grains are harvested and milled to make wheat flour. It has never been looked upon as having much value because it is so indigestible, but this is one of its virtues. The fact that bran is so indigestible means that when it is consumed there is a residue of material leaving the small bowel and entering the colon or large bowel. This retains water and helps to form a soft large stool which stimulates the muscles of the bowel and is easy to pass. That's the ideal picture but, as we now know, there are some significant problems with bran.

The first trials of bran in IBS were very effective and encouraged many doctors to recommend it as the answer. This initial enthusiasm was not maintained as more recent studies revealed that there was little overall benefit for IBS sufferers as a whole, though it can benefit some who mainly have constipation.

There are several types of bran depending upon the grain from which they are obtained. Wheat bran is the most common and the highest in fibre; oat bran is also popular and can help lower elevated blood cholesterol levels; and rice and soya bran contain less fibre than the others.

**Problems with bran**   There are a number of problems with bran, especially wheat bran, as listed below.

1 The indigestible fibre can be broken down or fermented by bacteria in the colon to produce a lot of gas. For some this may not be much of a problem but for others it can result in a lot of uncomfortable wind.
2 Bran contains a lot of phytic acid – a compound that blocks or interferes with the absorption of many minerals including calcium, magnesium, iron, zinc, copper and others. This may result in the person's diet being less nutritious rather than more so.
3 Quite a number of those with IBS are not able to eat wheat and other grains which for some unknown reason can aggravate their symptoms. This means that some sufferers are made worse by eating bran and are better off if they avoid it.

Some of these effects do diminish with time but many find that there is little help to their IBS when they take bran. Oat bran or just coarse oats may be a better type of fibre to take.

## Non-bran fibre-rich preparations

There are a number of medical fibre preparations that can help a sluggish bowel. Fibre-rich plants and seeds are used in these medical preparations, and they swell enormously when wet. Although they are not normal foods they can be very useful in the treatment of IBS and constipation. They include:

- Methylcellulose (Celevac) – a type of plant fibre.
- Sterculia (Normacol) – another sticky type of plant fibre.

- Ispaghula husk (Fybogel, Isogel and Regulan) – a sticky type of fibre.

- Grain fibre (Proctofibe and Trifyba) – unsuitable for those sensitive to grains.

With these bulk laxatives, it is important that you drink plenty of fluid mainly as water or fruit juice. Too much tea could worsen the constipation.

Also rather than over-rely on these added forms of fibre it is best to get as much fibre as you can from fruit, vegetables, nuts, seeds and grains. Some of these are particularly rich in the water-retaining types of fibre. Even so, not everyone can get all their fibre from foods alone and some supplement may be needed.

## Mineral salt preparations

These are a type of bulk laxative where the bulk is provided by water that is retained in the bowel not because of fibre but because of the presence of certain salts. Magnesium, sulphate and other salts, if taken in large amounts, are not fully absorbed from the gut, so they help to hold a certain amount of water in the colon and thereby act as a laxative.

An old and somewhat unfriendly preparation is Epsom Salts or magnesium sulphate. Magnesium hydroxide mixture is also available as a white liquid which is sometimes used for indigestion because of its acid-neutralizing properties. Other magnesium-rich preparations can be very useful as laxatives; they are very safe and effective, especially if combined with a high-fibre diet. This may be even more true for constipated women, particularly those with PMS because it is now known that many of them have a relative lack of this important essential mineral.

## Other bulk laxatives

**Lactulose**   This is an artificial, indigestible sugar which comes as a very sweet syrup. Like dietary fibre it arrives in the large bowel unchanged where the normal resident bacteria ferment it to produce some gas and lactic and acetic acids. These increase the bulk of the stool, soften it, and also stimulate regular gentle contraction of the bowel muscles, which may be useful for some.

## Stimulant laxatives

There are many drugs and natural chemicals that stimulate the bowel.

*Senna* is a powerful laxative derived from a Middle Eastern shrub.

It acts by stimulating the nerves that in turn control the muscles of the bowel wall. Prolonged or excessive use of senna over many years actually damages these same nerves resulting in a paralysis of the bowel. Senna should therefore only be used occasionally but it is a useful treatment for those with resistant constipation. Many herbal preparations contain senna and the same caution has to be observed with their use too.

*Cascara, rhubarb and aloes* are all old-fashioned, moderately effective laxatives that are derived from plant extracts.

*Danthron* is a similar stimulant laxative used in some medical preparations (such as Codalax, Co-Danthramer and Normax, among others). This compound has recently been reported as the cause of intestinal tumours in mice and rats, and it is not recommended for use on a prolonged basis.

*Bisacodyl and sodium picosulphate* are two drugs that also act as powerful bowel stimulants. They are used mainly for the elderly.

## Stool softeners

*Liquid paraffin* Perhaps the most well known but not the most advisable laxative, this tasteless oil is undigested and simply 'greases' the lower bowel. It is effective but not very safe, and prolonged use could interface with the absorption of the fat-soluble vitamins (A, D, E and K) as well as producing other health problems.

*Others* A number of chemical and stool softeners are used in some medical preparations (Co-Danthramer, Normax and others) usually with the stimulant laxative, Danthron. They are effective for some but useful mainly for the elderly.

## *Anti-diarrhoea preparations*

These drugs mainly work by inhibiting rather than by stimulating the nerves and muscles of the bowel, so that it is slowed down.

## Codeine and related compounds

Codeine is a popular anti-diarrhoea preparation which is derived from opium. In addition to its painkilling properties, like all similar drugs it is an effective treatment for diarrhoea. Codeine acts on the muscles of the gut sending those that pass food along the gut to sleep and curiously stimulating those that cut across the bowel. The slower passage along the bowel gives more time for water to be absorbed. While it causes few side-effects, it is not intended for prolonged regular use because dependency can develop.

Lomotil is the proprietary name of a similar preparation to codeine, while loperamide is another longer-acting similar drug. Most of these drugs have few side-effects if used carefully. They are mainly prescribed for acute diarrhoea but are sometimes used in IBS.

## Anti-wind drugs

*Charcoal* is an old and unfortunately not very effective treatment for excessive wind. Charcoal biscuits are almost only consumed by the elderly who were brought up in the belief that they work. In theory they could be quite effective, as charcoal has the ability to soak up certain gases and toxins that might be present in the gut as part of some people's IBS. However, it is difficult to imagine that charcoal taken by mouth would have much impact on what happens many hours or a day later in the colon. If you are desperate, it is perhaps worth considering and at least it is harmless.

*Bulking agents* As well as being used in constipation, these can sometimes help those with excessive wind. Methyl cellulose (Celevac) can bind with hydrogen sulphide (bad-eggs gas) and can act as a deodorizing agent.

## Anti-spasm drugs

The purpose of these drugs is to prevent the spasm of bowel muscles that is a feature of many patients' IBS.

*Mebeverine* (Colofac) relaxes overactive colon muscles, and it can be combined with a fibre supplement (Colven).

*Alverine* (Spasmonal) is another anti-spasmodic and it too can be combined with a fibre preparation (Alvercol).

### Atropine and related compounds

These are powerful old-fashioned drugs which originally were made from plant extracts. They block the nerves of the gut and elsewhere, and are still used in some older preparations. They are effective at a price; side-effects include a dry mouth, urinary difficulties, blurred vision, flushing, dry skin and palpitations. They are not suitable for the elderly or for those with glaucoma.

### Peppermint oil

This is one home remedy that really does have some science behind it, because the oil from peppermint can help to relax the muscles of the colon. It can be taken in a capsule (Colpermin and Mintec) that delays the release of the oil until it reaches the end of the small bowel. Side-effects are few but occasionally allergic reactions do occur.

## Drugs that help stimulate the muscles of the gut

In more recent times, a number of drugs have been developed that act by stimulating the muscles of the upper gut. They are useful in situations where there is a disturbance of the oesophagus or stomach with symptoms of excessive wind (upwards), indigestion, and excessive fullness after meals.

These drugs include cisapride (Alimix and Prepulsid), metoclopramide (Maxolon and Gastromax) and domperidone (Motilium). They may occasionally be used in those with IBS who also have the above symptoms. All these drugs can have side-affects especially metoclopramide which can cause drowsiness, diarrhoea, the production of a milky fluid from women's breasts and disturbance of the nervous system – mainly in the elderly. They are powerful drugs to be used with caution.

## A final word

The intention of all these drugs is to control symptoms and not to treat any underlying problem. They are perfectly worthy but their effectiveness has been rather overplayed. You may have been prescribed one or more of these preparations and found them only to be partially successful. They are perfectly all right to use in the short term, but many are unsuitable for long-term use. Indeed while they are being taken, the patient and doctor or other therapist should be looking at what else can be done to help solve the problem, particularly in the way of dietary change and stress control.

# 10

# The role of stress in IBS

While a certain amount of stress may be good for us, since it tends to keep us mentally on the ball, there comes a point when stress can be overwhelming. Feeling stressed out for any length of time can take its toll on a person, both physically and mentally. It has long been medically acknowledged over the years that stress can affect the digestive process. Additionally, when we are under considerable emotional and psychological stress, it is possible that we are more likely to develop food intolerances. Often the stress persists, the symptoms become chronic, or the individual may be passed off as neurotic or a hypochondriac, and things go from bad to worse. In-effective treatment, or inadequate belief in the physical nature of our symptoms, often contributes further to our stress. There is firm medical evidence to support the fact that stress aggravates symptoms.

## Elizabeth's story

Elizabeth Saunders is an 18-year-old student from Buckingham-shire. She had been suffering with her symptoms since childhood and felt that they were ruining her life. Although she has overcome her symptoms now, she still has a lot of upset about her treatment since she was young.

'I started to suffer when I was seven years old. My tummy used to get very bloated and very very painful. I had constant wind and severe constipation. I had spasms that left me severely prostrated with the pain, and on a really bad day you could actually see my in-testines as they were so swollen. The list was endless. My family didn't believe that I was really suffering because my doctor told them that I was just trying to avoid school. I was told that I was mentally disturbed, which after a while I started to believe since there just didn't seem to be a solution.

'As a child, I was allowed to drink Coca Cola for a treat with my Sunday dinner. Little did we know that I was highly allergic to it and as soon as I had one sip, I would be in agony. My father would get really cross because he thought I was just trying to get out of school on Monday. I soon gained a reputation as a trouble maker, which I supposed you might call the self-fulfilling prophecy, as I began to live up to it. I wanted help and was told I was bad, so I had to do something to make people listen. I would take at least five days to recover from one glass of Coke and so the vicious circle continued.

'All my doctor did was prescribe painkillers and laxatives. He told me to eat more wheat, and to stop imagining things, and eventually he referred me to a psychiatrist. I spent a week in hospital at one point, and have been in and out of hospital for tests for years now.

'I should mention that things became much worse when I was a teenager, as I developed severe PMS and became violent and impossible to say the least. This, on top of the problems with my tummy, became unbearable. I was desperate. I had no one to turn to and so depended on alcohol to solve my problems.

'I heard about the WNAS through a friend. The doctor at the WNAS clinic explained how certain foods and drinks might be aggravating my symptoms. I cut out all tea, coffee, alcohol, fizzy drinks, cigarettes and goods that contain gluten – like wheat, oats, barley and rye. I replaced all this with a healthy diet and drank plenty of water. I also took up Yoga, to calm my shattered nerves.

'With the genuine support and help from the WNAS I have discovered that alcohol makes me violent and wheat makes me very depressed. Both affect my tummy adversely. I now also take Linusit Gold every day which, together with extra magnesium supplements, helps to keep me regular. I found, too, that "Optivite", the multi vitamin and mineral supplement for women, keeps things ticking along nicely. Sticking to this simple diet has made me into a new person!

'The WNAS has been marvellous for me. What they have to offer is very empowering to the patients, as they can help us to help ourselves. I have finally got control of my life again, and I can honestly say that the WNAS was the first big step there. I have no more bowel problems and no more PMS either. I feel strongly that people should not be left to suffer in silence. Doctors and everyone in general should be better educated so that we know the genuine signs to look for. I am now old enough to put things right for myself, but nothing will make up for the time I missed off school and the misery I felt as a child. Adults and doctors are in a position of trust, and there to protect and help children, not to ruin young lives through ignorance and lack of compassion.'

# Life in the fast lane

In the nerve-racking 1990s, more and more of us have had to cope with real problems. The recession in the UK has claimed many victims who have, perhaps for the first time in their lives, experienced harsh financial difficulties. Women in particular often have more on their hands than they might have had only one or two generations ago. As well as having the family and home to look after, they often have to work outside the home to make ends meet, without having an extended family to fall back on. When time is short and energy levels are low, you can see the attraction that convenience food has over home cooking. As fast food inevitably contains fewer nutrients than wholesome food, many of us are not meeting our bodies' needs on a day-to-day basis. The body eventually tells us that all is not well by producing symptoms of one sort or another. In some it may be migraine headaches, or poor skin quality, while in others it may be symptoms of IBS.

On the other side of the coin, while those who work long hours often daydream about having more spare time, being unemployed can be equally stressful all by itself, without considering any of the other stresses that have to be faced as part of everyday living.

A large number of patients we see with IBS have experienced an overdose of stress, which they acknowledge has made their symptoms worse. Many of us have the amazing ability to cope with near tragedy or near disaster. It is sometimes not until the dust has settled after the event that we then subconsciously let ourselves fall apart. During stressful periods we often let our diet slip, and eat processed snacks which tend to be high in calories, and low in fibre and essential nutrients. Consuming insufficient nutrients to meet the body's demand and drinking too much tea, coffee and alcohol, can be the final straw, or possibly bring on the symptoms of IBS.

## Why me?

You might well reasonably ask why it is that some people cope with stress and maintain their health while others physically crumble. First, remember that, nutritionally speaking, we are all the product of several generations. Some, therefore, clearly have advantages over others. Another important factor that should be considered is our ability to confront problems and deal with them, without feeling too overwhelmed even if it involves taking professional advice.

The old saying 'a problem shared is a problem halved' is very true. Talking through something you are worried about with a friend, family member or counsellor can help you to see your way through the fog. You may be surprised by the number of people who get real satisfaction out of helping others. So don't be afraid to open up. Several studies have shown that psychotherapy and counselling do help some people with IBS. A Swedish study using simple supportive counselling, given over a course of eight sessions to a group of patients with IBS, produced significantly reduced symptoms within three months, when compared to a group who did not receive therapy.

## Hypnotherapy and relaxation

Hypnotherapy has been used in trials to treat symptoms of IBS. One particular study, conducted in Manchester by Whorwell and his colleagues, used a combination of education about the working of the gut and its muscles, half-hour sessions of hypnotherapy of decreasing frequency, and where appropriate the use of bulk laxatives. The hypnotherapy induced a state of relaxation and an improved sense of control over bowel muscle function. Encouraging and supportive comments were also made when the individual was under hypnosis.

Many of the 50 patients in this study did well. The overall success rate for the group, after an average time of 18 months from starting treatment, was a commendable 84 per cent. Further analysis allowed some conclusions to be drawn about who was likely to do well and who was not. Those with painless diarrhoea, those with mainly pain without much disturbance in bowel habit, and older patients aged 50 or more responded less well in this study. For young patients with classic symptoms the success rate was 100 per cent.

Clearly there is a substantial value to this approach but because bulk laxatives were used in addition to the hypnotherapy it is not possible to be certain which part of the regime actually helped them to overcome their symptoms or whether it was the combination of approaches.

Once you have identified the source of your stress, apart from making a plan – with or without the help of a counsellor – to overcome the problem or circumstances in which you find yourself, you are bound to benefit from making time to eat well, take regular exercise, creating time to relax every day, even if it is just for 15 minutes, and to get as much fresh air as you can.

If you cultivate the ability to stand 'outside yourself' and look at your problems from an exterior point of view, and consider circumstances that could be much worse, you may well see things in a different light.

# 11

# Relaxation and exercise

Why does hypnotherapy and relaxation work? It might be because they genuinely cause an improvement in the way the bowel functions and, in particular, in the way in which the muscles of the gut wall work in an efficient and co-ordinated fashion. An alternative explanation is that this type of approach is effective because it makes the person less sensitive to, or more tolerant of, the disturbance in the function of their bowels. Perhaps both are relevant.

Stress and relaxation are at two opposite ends of the spectrum. When they are in balance all is well, but when stress outweighs relaxation, symptoms often develop. Our modern lifestyle is far from relaxed. We should therefore consciously protect ourselves from excess stress by learning relaxation techniques which, unlike stress, do not come naturally, and above all make the time to practise them.

Basic relaxation techniques, exercise, yoga, massage, autogenic training, creative visualization, biofeedback and heat are all ways in which we can reduce the stress and tension that aggravate symptoms. Let us look at these regimes individually and assess their merits.

## *Basic relaxation techniques*

Learning to release tension from tensed muscles is an acquired skill. However, once learned, it can be practised at any time, requires only space and time, and is free of charge. Rather than focusing on the outside world and the problems that it brings, you will need to learn to tune in to your body and become sensitive to its tensions.

Even if you have never had any instruction in basic relaxation techniques, what is involved is quite simple. You will need to wear some loose clothing, and find a warm space, where you can remain uninterrupted. Either lie down on a mat, on a soft carpet, or on a bed. Then place a pillow under your head and relax your arms and your jaw. Take a few slow deep breaths before you begin, and then concentrate on relaxing your muscles, starting with the toes on one foot, and then the other, gradually working your way slowly up your body. Tense each group of muscles first, and then relax them, taking care to breathe deeply as you relax. When you reach your head and your face feels relaxed, remain in the relaxed position for about 15 minutes. Then allow yourself to come to gradually. If you are keen on music, you can try practising this relaxation technique while calming music is playing in the background.

## *Yoga*

For thousands of years, yoga has been practised throughout the world. It works on the principle of bringing about a harmonious balance between your mind, body and soul. It is particularly effective at helping to relieve stress and thus stress-related conditions. It is best to attend a yoga class to get started, and then to practise the postures at home on a regular basis. There are many good books on yoga and there are now a few yoga videos which you may find helpful.

## *Massage*

We often subconsciously touch or rub a painful area in an attempt to bring about relief. Massage is a term used to describe a fairly ancient art of healing by touch. There are now several different massage techniques, but essentially massage is designed to heal, relieve tension, improve circulation and help the body to rid itself of toxins. Massage can also relieve pain by stimulating the production of endorphins, the body's own painkillers, and by blocking out the transmission of pain messages by increasing the sensory input to the brain. It can be administered by a qualified masseuse, a partner or a friend, or alternatively you can learn to self-massage. Just rubbing your abdomen in a clockwise direction with some almond oil, and possibly a few drops of aromatherapy oil, can be very soothing and can help to ease spasmodic constipation.

If you enjoy being massaged, you might enjoy learning how to massage by following a short course. Teaming up with another can be the cheapest way to get a regular massage. Again, there are a number of good books written on the subject.

## Creative visualization, self-hypnosis, autogenic training and biofeedback

These are all methods of stimulating the subconscious mind to heal the body. It is thought that the subconscious can be influenced by suggestion and imagination, hence the placebo response that we sometimes hear about. As individuals have differing likes and dislikes, it is comforting to know that we have a choice of therapy, in order to achieve our end objective.

Creative visualization is probably one of the easiest and most pleasant of pastimes. It really just involves day-dreaming in a structured way. Choose a scene that you would like to be part of, and spirit yourself there in your mind. The skill you will gradually acquire involves blocking out everything else, and being able to be in your desired scene, feeling warm, calm and relaxed.

The technique of self-hypnosis can help to bring about a feeling of calmness and mental agility. It is a system of implanting positive messages which have a therapeutic value. Half an hour each day can leave you feeling refreshed and in a positive mood.

Autogenic training is a method designed to tap into the body's own in-built powers of self-healing. It consists of repeating six different commands slowly in sequence until you reach a semi-hypnotic state. The end result is a much more relaxed and positive you – and requires only half an hour or so three times per week initially.

Biofeedback is another relaxation technique. Here you are linked to a biofeedback machine, or more recently, a Relaxometer. Reaching a deep state of relaxation has been shown to influence blood pressure levels and brainwave patterns.

All of these and many more relaxation techniques can be learned at specialist centres throughout the country. It may be worth investing time on a few dark winter evenings to learn to outsmart the stresses and strains of daily life.

It is worth trying out a few techniques before you decide on the one for you. When you find a workable method, that has a positive effect on you both physically and mentally, you will have the incentive to practise on a regular basis.

## The value of exercise

The positive value of exercise should not be underestimated. It is a fact that exercise is of general benefit to people of all ages, as it is necessary for optimum function, structure and preservation of muscles, bones, joints and the heart. Regular exercise can extend and improve the quality of an active life, and plays a vital part in the prevention of many chronic conditions. Apart from helping to keep your body ticking over, gentle aerobic exercises will encourage the release of the brain chemicals called endorphins, which help you raise your mood, alleviate depression and reduce sensitivity to pain. If you have been experiencing severe symptoms, and your mood has been subdued as a result, try doing some gentle exercise to start with, and build yourself up to three or four good sessions of aerobic exercise a week.

Exercise is a very personal thing. You are not competing with anyone, so you will need to choose the type of exercise you enjoy, whether it is swimming, jogging or a work-out in front of the video. Build your stamina up gradually. If you have any health problems apart from your IBS symptoms, and you have not exercised for some time, you should go along to your doctor for a physical check-up before starting.

## *Heat*

The warmth of the sun or even a hot-water bottle can help to relax tense muscles, and thus ease away pain. If you experience severe tummy cramps, try lying face down on a soft surface, with a hot-water bottle or a heat pad under the painful part. If you cannot afford yourself the luxury of going to bed, you could try placing a thermal heat pad inside your skirt or your trousers, while you continue with your chores. These 'hand-sized' chemically activated heat pads can be re-used over and over again, and are small enough to be carried around in your handbag or your briefcase. They are available by mail order, and the details are on page 248.

Whichever therapy you decide to opt for, make sure you enjoy it, and practise it regularly. You must make time to pamper yourself a little, and regard the time spent as an investment. It will undoubtedly pay dividends in the long term as it is likely to speed up the healing process.

# 12

# A new start

You can now pause for breath, as you have reached the end of the theory section about what underlies IBS symptoms. From reading Part One, you should be more aware of what is happening to your body, and have had a glimpse of the possibility of leading a symptom-free life. You may be feeling sceptical about the workability of the plan, or you may be wondering whether you will be able to cope with a new way of eating. The vast majority of our patients felt the same way initially, but the thing that they all had in common is that they were willing to follow the recommendations and give the programme a chance to work.

The Diet Plan lasts for ten weeks, and contains nine specific stages. You will need to make sure that you have a period of ten weeks during which you won't need to stay in a hotel, so that you can prepare food for yourself. The mental attitude required is that of embarking on an adventure. Try to feel positive about following the plan each day, and stick rigidly to the instructions. This way you will only have to do the experiment once.

We very much hope that Part Two will pave the way to your recovery. On page 96 we have provided a blank chart for you to construct your own programme. As you read through the sections that apply to you in Chapters 13, 14 and 15, you will need to make a note of the specific recommendations and variations that you feel are most applicable to your symptoms. These then dovetail in with the instructions given in Phases 1 to 8 of the Plan.

Once you have made a start on the diet, you will need to complete the daily chart, which can be found on page 100. This will give you an invaluable running record to refer back to as you go along.

We wish you good luck with your experiment, and hope that you will soon discover exactly what has been causing your symptoms.

*part two*
# The solution

# 13

# The voyage of discovery

## Ann's story

When Ann Saxton contacted the WNAS she had been sick for nine years. She was 24 years old, recently married and lived in London.

'A journalist friend of mine, who had recently written about the WNAS suggested I contact them for help. I had been suffering with IBS since I was 15 years old, plus I had severe recurring cystitis and PMS. Over the years I had been seen not only by my GP, but also by several different specialists in London. I had had numerous tests, none of which showed any major abnormalities. I tried all sorts of medication including the contraceptive pill, and all the usual preparations used for IBS. None of them seemed to help at all and so I was told by one and all that I would have to learn to live with my symptoms as there was nothing more that could be done for me.

'The quality of my life suffered greatly as a result of all the symptoms from which I continually seemed to suffer. Fortunately my husband is an understanding person, because I certainly tried his patience.

'When I began the programme written for me by the WNAS I wasn't sure I could follow it through. I had been a wholefood vegetarian for many years, and ate lots of wholewheat products. The basic diet initially suggested involved cutting out grains like wheat, oats, barley and rye, as well as cutting down on tea, coffee and salt.

'As I was feeling so ill, I decided to try the diet, even though it was dramatically different from that which I was used to. I continued to eat seitan, a macrobiotic food from Japan, until I realized that it too was made of wheat. I was also using lots of tamari (soy sauce) in my cooking, until it was pointed out that this had a high salt and yeast content.

'I felt dramatically different within the first month, and within three months I was feeling tremendous. Virtually all my symptoms had gone completely. I was free of IBS, my cystitis had cleared up and the PMS was gone too.

'I found it hard to believe that the diet, the supplements and the

exercise had been the total solution. So I went back to eating carbohydrates, and left out the vitamin and mineral pills. Lo and behold,
back came all those ghastly symptoms. I quickly reverted to the new
diet and the supplements and managed to control the symptoms
again. I am undoubtedly convinced now, and know that I will have to
maintain my new diet in order to remain symptom free, at least in
the short term.'

Unless you are reading this book in order to understand someone
else's IBS, we assume that you have IBS symptoms and have
reached the point where you are ready to make an investment and a
few sacrifices in order to restore your health and improve the quality
of your life. As long as you have no other major health problems, the
right programme should help you to achieve these objectives.

We usually associate 'diets' with weight loss, and improved
appearance rather than increased health. Traditionally, dieters go
on diets year in and year out, in what's known as the yo-yo syndrome. People are usually motivated at the time of starting a diet by
the desire to be slimmer, but in weak moments their enthusiasm
often wanes. Finding a diet to suit your body, and one that will help
you back to health, is quite a different matter. If you have really been
suffering with your symptoms, you will no doubt be motivated to
keep them at bay. However, as you will have gathered from some of
the stories from other sufferers, people do stray from the diet once
their symptoms are under control. It seems to be a fact related to
human nature! Everyone has a short memory when it comes to pain
and discomfort, which is probably just as well.

Once you are armed with the knowledge about what your body
likes and dislikes in relation to your symptoms, you will be able to
judge in the long term what you can and cannot tolerate. In our experience, when patients 'go off the rails', as they put it, and symptoms recur as a result, they do not need to be told to tighten up their
regime. So during the process of the 'experiment' you are about to
undertake, you will be getting to know your body and its require-
ments, maybe for the first time ever.

The secret to success is getting the diet right for you. Sometimes
just missing one factor can throw the whole thing off course. For
some, finding the right kind of diet can be a relatively simple pro-
cedure, while for others it can be a good deal more tricky. Belinda
Lavery is a patient who springs to mind at this point.

## _____ Belinda's story _____

Belinda is a single 32-year-old who came to the clinic on the recommendation of a friend. She had been suffering with severe bowel problems for two years which were causing her extreme distress. Her work life was affected and her social life was non-existent as a result.

'Looking back I realize that my symptoms began at about the time that my relationship ended with my boyfriend. We had been together for two years, and I found it very difficult to cope with the break-up. Although outwardly I went through the motions of life, it obviously affected me physically. I began to have severe episodes of bloating, and constipation every day, with extreme abdominal pain. I even found it difficult to sit down at work. Each day by the evening I was in so much pain, I could only go to bed and wait for the pain to subside. I felt awfully drained and lost quite a bit of weight, which I could ill afford to do.

'My GP thought it was a hormonal problem originally as my periods disappeared at the same time. He prescribed some drugs to bring on my periods, which they did, but as the other problems persisted, I stopped taking them. I was referred to the hospital for tests, including small bowel enema, ultra sound and X-rays, and in November 1992 I was diagnosed as having IBS, and told to go on a high-fibre diet. The hospital doctor told me there was no known cure, and when I asked in desperation what I could do as I was still in constant pain, and with a redundant wardrobe, due to the swelling, he said I would have to buy bigger clothes. I was very shocked and angry by his unsympathetic response.

'So a vicious circle began. I took painkillers, which brought on severe constipation and distress, which could only be relieved by laxatives. My doctor prescribed Colpermin, to make eating easier, but this only brought me out in a rash and the list of possible side-effects was quite alarming.

'I sought help from my mother's homoeopath at this point and took a remedy called Ignatia. The transformation was remarkable, I was actually able to eat normally without any pain, and my periods returned. However, the change was short lived, and I was virtually back to square one within three weeks.

'In May 1993 I went along to the WNAS clinic at the suggestion of a friend who had been treated successfully by them. When I went for my first appointment I must admit that I felt sceptical. I couldn't imagine that diet alone would be the solution to this severe problem.

I was put on to a basic diet, asked to keep daily symptoms charts and was seen fortnightly for a review. While I did have some good days, I still had more bad days. I was given an amended set of dietary recommendations to follow at each visit. After three months and very little change I was on the verge of giving up, when I was told that, in addition to excluding the foods we had so far, I should also leave out rice, corn, potatoes and bananas. It was also suggested that I should take Linusit Gold with my cereals and extra magnesium at night to relieve the constipation. To my utter amazement, my symptoms calmed down. The constipation was no longer a problem and the pain and bloating subsided.

'I now live on a relatively restricted diet, but I manage well and am happy on it. I have the odd bad day when I stray from the diet, although nothing like the 'beached whale' of two years ago. I have gained a few pounds in weight, and at least I feel that I can get on with my life now and look to the future, rather than dreading each day. I am very pleased I followed my friend's advice.'

---

We cannot promise you that going on the Diet Plan will be a picnic. While things may go very smoothly, and your symptoms may 'vanish' within a few weeks, you should prepare yourself for a few setbacks, and then you won't feel too disappointed. As setbacks often bring on symptoms, you may even hit a few low points, like Belinda did, and feel like giving up. Along with thousands of others, she is glad that she persevered, and you will be too. Whatever you do, see it through to the end. With our patients, it is easy for us to help them over the hurdles as they present themselves. But because you will be left to your own devices, it is important to be forewarned. You will need to keep accurate daily records of your symptoms, and of your diet if you deviate from the diet suggested. You will find the charts on page 100. Do not forget to complete them, because they are as important as the diet itself. They will prove invaluable for review purposes as time progresses.

You will see by looking through the diet section that it is split up into specific sections relating to different groups of foods and drinks. You *must* stick to the rules of the diet rigidly, if you are to come out at the end with an accurate evaluation. The first two weeks are the basic diet, devoid of most of the common foods and drinks that trigger symptoms. If you suffer with constipation, and are still constipated after the first two weeks, you will need to repeat one of the first two weeks, making three weeks in total on the basic sheet.

We have tried to make the diet as interesting and nutritious as possible. There are many delicious recipes in the recipe sections, which correspond with the menus. If you are working, or cooking for one, you may not wish to go to the bother of preparing so many meals for yourself, or you simply may not have the time. For this reason, we have included some Fast Options, which you will find just before the menus for each section.

Again, we must stress the importance of reading Part One of this book before going on the actual diet itself. It is essential that you consider what may lie behind your symptoms, and indeed whether they need any further investigation, before you start on the diet. We cannot promise that it will be plain sailing, but we can more or less guarantee that this will be a voyage of discovery, the result of which we hope will improve your understanding of the needs of your body, and set you free to lead your life.

# Tips to overcome symptoms

Your symptoms will dictate which of the following tips you will find helpful. Read through the sections that apply to you and make specific notes as you go along. Your final test will need to be incorporated into the diet you follow, certainly for the first two weeks while you are following the basic diet.

## Ways to reduce your constipation

- **Eat plenty of fibre-rich foods**   This means all fruit and vegetables, nuts and seeds, some cereals – brown rice, sweetcorn (maize), buckwheat, sago and tapioca. Take care, as some of these foods might make other symptoms worse especially if you have bloating and wind.

- **Take a fibre supplement**   This can be from your doctor or from a health food shop. Good supplements include those containing ispaghula (Fybogel), sterculia (Normacol), linseeds (Linusit Gold) and, when tolerated, coarse oats. They are all highly water retentive and can be very effective especially when combined with other measures to stimulate movement through the gut.

- **Ensure a good intake of fluid**   This is very important if you are elderly or you are taking a fibre supplement.

- **Avoid wheat, oats, barley and rye**   and all foods containing them. This is a major change to your diet and you will need to refer to Chapter 25.

- **Cut down or stop your consumption of tea**   Limit yourself to two cups of weak tea a day.

- **Drink one or two cups of coffee instead of tea**   This may act as a laxative for some. The stimulating effect appears to take about 60 minutes before it is noticeable.

- **Have a cigarette!**   Yes, if you are already a smoker, you may be aware that a few puffs – especially first thing in the morning or after your main meal – can help you open your bowels. This is no recommendation to start smoking and no excuse not to give up but if you are going to smoke you might as well use it to help your bowels along.

- **Take some magnesium**   This seems particularly relevant if you have constipation without diarrhoea; have severe slow transit constipation (two or less motions per week); have premenstrual problems or have fatigue as a major problem. Magnesium may benefit these conditions in particular. A safe dose is 200–400 mg of magnesium a day. Doses higher than this can be taken but not on a regular basis without your doctor's approval. Almost any type of magnesium will do. Magnesium oxide, gluconate and chelate are available from health food shops and tend to be quite gentle. Magnesium hydroxide (in the form of a white liquid) and sulphate (in the form of crystals) are much more dramatic in their effect. A good time to take magnesium is last thing at night because this will tend to help you to open your bowels the following morning. All green vegetables are an excellent source of this mineral.

- **Remember that regular exercise can only help**   Try exercising three times a week. Choose something that you enjoy or have enjoyed in the past and that you can do regularly.

- **Avoid stressful situations whenever possible**   Yoga is an excellent way of relaxing and helps you to tolerate stress better. Listening to music, going for a walk, eating a good meal (diet permitting) or just enjoying the company of family and friends are all useful and effective ways of reducing tension.

- **Set aside time for your bowels**   Often it is easier for some people to open their bowels at certain times of the day. For many with constipation and IBS this may be in the morning on rising or just after eating breakfast. If this is the case then try to make arrangements so that you are not disturbed. Take the phone off the hook, make sure the kids have left for school and that no one is going to call. It may be helpful to have a hot drink or if you are a smoker a puff of that cigarette. Perhaps an early morning jog is the stimulus your bowel needs. Find out by trial and error what your bowels need to function smoothly and with a regular daily pattern.

- **Take a laxative**  Choose from those given in Chapter 9. If you need advice, ask the pharmacist at your local chemist or speak to your doctor. In our experience, a good combination is to combine a fibre supplement (like Linusit Gold) and magnesium, taking them on a regular daily basis, with a more powerful laxative, such as senna or a prescribed preparation, taken once or twice a week, if needed. Never exceed the stated dosage of these preparations.

  If you are taking drug medication that might aggravate your constipation then check this with your doctor. And certainly see him or her if you have any painful condition that makes it difficult for you to go to the toilet.

It can take a while before the full benefit of these treatments and changes may be experienced. As a rule, fibre supplements and laxatives will have an effect within a week or two. The exception to this is magnesium, which might take several weeks or even two or three months before it has its maximum effect.

The dietary changes outlined here can take up to four weeks before they achieve a beneficial result. You will also need to make some changes to your lifestyle as outlined and to establish a regular exercise regime.

# Ways to reduce the pain of IBS

- **Tackle the factors that cause or aggravate constipation**  See Chapter 5 page 30. This alone may be enough for many with IBS.

- **Avoid foods that you know or strongly suspect aggravate any of your IBS symptoms**  including diarrhoea and wind.

- **Avoid painkillers that contain codeine or related compounds**  Their main side-effect is constipation which is likely to make things worse in the long run. Paracetamol is more likely to be suitable but should only be taken as a short-term measure.

- **Ask your doctor to prescribe a medicine with anti-spasm properties**  Colpermin, based on peppermint, can help relax tense gut muscles.

- **Try taking a regular daily supplement of magnesium**  This is essential if you are constipated despite making changes to your diet. Magnesium in the form of amino acid chelate, gluconate or oxide seems particularly appropriate. A reasonable dose is 200 mg two or three times a day. Diarrhoea is the only likely side-effect of taking too much.

- **Never ignore the urge to open your bowels!** If you hear the call, go, or be prepared to suffer the consequences.

- **Relax** Even if you are in pain, try to relax. Sit down, lie down or go to sleep if you can. Yoga, self-hypnosis, listening to some of your favourite music can all help. Find out what works for you.

- **Try using a hot-water bottle or heat pad** Applying heat to a painful and troubled abdomen can help to soothe the pain.

- **Have a massage** Gentle massage of the lower back can help to ease the pain for some, and sometimes a very light massage of the abdomen can be helpful too. Always do this in a clockwise movement, the direction of flow through the colon.

- **Treat any painful condition affecting the anus** This may mean seeing your doctor to get treatment for your piles. Glycerine suppositories are a simple way of helping to overcome the constipation due to painful anal conditions.

- **Try a cup of Rooibosch tea** made from the South African red bush – Eleven O'clock variety has been shown to relax the muscles.

- **Try a homoeopathic remedy** Choose colocynth for abdominal cramps; nux vomica for painful constipation; calc carb for abdominal bloating with wind; and phosphoric acid for painless diarrhoea and fatigue. Most homoeopathic remedies are available from local chemists and health food shops or from specialist suppliers.

- **See your doctor** if your pain is long standing, severe, if it changes, or if it is associated with feelings of depression or anxiety. Sometimes a small dose of anti-depressant drug can have useful painkilling properties.

It is quite likely that a number of other foods and herbs have relaxing effects on the gut. You may want to consult a qualified herbalist who can prescribe some herbs based on your specific symptoms. Homoeopathic remedies can also be a useful way of reducing pain. These simple, usually natural compounds are given as a tiny dose which can be repeated several times a day, but, like many other therapies, they are not always effective. Choose from the following:

- Colocynthis – useful for abdominal pain with diarrhoea that is worse after eating.
- Calc Carb – taken for abdominal bloating, wind and loss of appetite.
- Nux Vomica – a remedy for constipation, with painful and unproductive attempts to open the bowels.
- Phosphoric acid – used for diarrhoea usually without much pain but associated with weakness.

## Ways to reduce diarrhoea

- **Consider avoiding wheat, oats, barley and rye**

- **Consider avoiding milk, yoghurt, cream and cheese** Other foods containing these foods or lactose (milk sugar) should also be avoided.

- **Eat moderate-sized meals and eat every two to three hours** This will help not to overburden your digestive system.

- **Eat slowly and chew your food well** Doing so may give your stomach and digestive system a much better chance to digest your food properly.

- **Adjust your fat intake** Generally it is a good idea for many to ensure that there is a moderate amount of fat in each main meal.

- **Stop or reduce your intake of coffee including decaffeinated brands** Consider drinking ordinary tea. This can slow the passage of food through the gut in about 50 per cent of people. Cut down on hot drinks if you think that this is a factor too.

- **Avoid excessive use of the artificial sweetener Sorbitol** Watch out for 'sugar-free' chewing gum and mints.

- **Avoid spicy foods, if they upset you** In theory, however, taking a large amount of chilli and other hot spices might slow the gut down and help diarrhoea.

- **Reduce or stop smoking** Try to pace yourself between cigarettes so that you gradually smoke fewer each day.

- **Reduce or stop drinking alcohol** Try to cut down to no more than three drinks a week initially.

- **If you suspect that a drug you are taking might be causing your diarrhoea, discuss this with your doctor or
specialist** A change of drug therapy may be necessary.

- **Try taking some strong yeast-free vitamin B complex** A
high dose providing 50–100 mg of most of the B vitamins including
vitamin B3 or nicotinamide is recommended as a daily dose. This
should not be taken without your doctor's approval if you are
known to be anaemic, have recently lost weight or have had
stomach or bowel surgery. Those with a high alcohol intake or
diarrhoea following antibiotic usage or following gastroenteritis
are particularly likely to benefit.

- **Avoid stress** (see Chapter 10).

If these tips are going to be helpful then some improvement should
be noticeable within four weeks. If this is not the case, then you
should check with your doctor.

## *What your doctor has on offer*

If you have not already seen your doctor about your diarrhoea then
you should consider doing so, especially if you have lost weight, are
aged over 50, or if the above tips have not proved helpful. Your
doctor can consider the following avenues:

1 Examination and investigations to look for a cause of the diarrhoea
   and assess the likelihood of nutritional deficiencies. Blood tests
   for anaemia and measurement of vitamin B, iron and zinc are
   widely available.
2 X-ray of the bowel using a barium meal or barium enema. Barium
   is a heavy inert mineral provided in the form of a liquid which
   shows up as dense white on X-ray and allows a good impression of
   the bowel and its lining to be obtained.
3 Endoscopy of the bowel. This is an examination of the gut, upper
   or lower, obtained by passing a sophisticated flexible telescope
   through it. This allows a close inspection of the lining of the bowel,
   and is particularly good for diagnosing inflammation of the bowel.
   Samples or biopsies from the gut lining can also be taken for
   further examination.
4 Arrange for a stool examination. This is a useful way to look for
   parasite infections if they are suspected, for blood in the stool and
   for an excess of undigested fat. If the diarrhoea is due to poor
   digestion and not straightforward IBS, this may show up as an

excess of fat in the stool. In fact, any cause of persistent diarrhoea can lead to a degree of difficulty in the digestion of fat and might then lead to mild nutritional deficiencies.

5 Prescribe a drug. Loperamide (Motilin) slows the passage of material along the gut, increases the amount of water absorbed by the gut and increases the tone of the anal muscles. Codeine phosphate is an old-fashioned drug derived from opium and, if taken in small doses, is relatively free from side-effects. Sodium cromoglycate (Nalcrom capsules) is an anti-allergy preparation used in spray form in the treatment of asthma. It can also be used in the form of capsules taken by mouth for those with true food allergies. One trial in Australia found that it also benefited eight out of 20 patients with diarrhoea due to IBS in whom food allergy had not originally been suspected. This preparation is worth considering as it has very few side-effects, but it is expensive, although it is available on the NHS.

6 Prescribe a vitamin supplement. As mentioned earlier, certain nutritional deficiencies can occur in association with diarrhoea. It may be appropriate for your doctor to give you some strong vitamin B complex or multivitamins and this will depend upon the results of appropriate investigations. Some standard UK NHS vitamin B and multivitamin preparations are not strong enough for the correction of severe nutritional deficiencies.

# Choosing your options

In an ideal world, it would be nice if you could press a button on this page and your personal diet options would appear. Unfortunately, the task will be a little more laborious for you, as you will need to select the options according to your symptoms. This is why the theory in Part One is so valuable.

We have designed the diet to be universal. In other words, it is suitable for all sufferers of IBS, no matter whether they have constipation, diarrhoea, pain, wind, or bloating as their main symptom. Because of this, there are variations that you have to follow according to your individual symptoms. In addition, it is obviously sensible to avoid any foods or drinks that you already know upset you, or which aggravate your symptoms in any way.

You will need to read through the following sections that apply to you, and make notes as you go through them to add to your list. A natural progression from the tips on overcoming the major IBS symptoms, is to look at dietary do's and don'ts.

## The basic diet – the first two weeks

The guidelines for the first two weeks are general, and must be superseded by the recommendations for your individual symptoms.

### *General guidelines for Phase One*

**Avoid completely**

Any foods or drinks that contain any of the following:

Wheat in any form, including bread, cakes, biscuits, pastry, pizza
Oats, barley, rye, or corn including maize and cornstarch
Potatoes
All citrus fruit, including oranges, grapefruit, satsumas, lemons
Chocolate, chocolate drinks, cola-based drinks
Sweets, popcorn and mints
Peanuts
Yeast-rich foods, including yeast extract, Marmite, Oxo, Knorr and

other stock cubes, vinegar and pickled food, chutneys, piccalilli,
sauces or condiments containing vinegar
Alcohol

## Food additives to avoid

While you cannot completely avoid food additives, it is best to avoid
those with some type of colouring and preservatives that are known
to aggravate allergies, and in some cases smelly wind. Whenever
possible avoid the following:

E102 Tartrazine
E104 Quinoline Yellow
E110 Sunset Yellow FCF or Orange Yellow S
E122 Carmoisine or Azorubine
E123 Amaranth
E124 Ponceau 4R or Cochineal Red A
E127 Erythrosine BS
E131 Patent Blue V
E132 Indigo Carmine or Indigotine
E142 Green S or Acid Brilliant
      Green BS or Lissamine Green
E151 Black PN or Brilliant Black BN
E180 Pigment Rubine or Lithol Rubine BK
E220–227 Sulphites

## What you can consume in moderation

Small amounts of sugar or honey
No more than two cups of tea and two cups of coffee a day
Nuts, excluding peanuts
Beans, as long as they don't give you symptoms of wind and bloating
Lentils, soya products, including soya milk and yoghurt
Peas and seeds
Root vegetables
Animal fats
Salt and black pepper

## What you can consume freely

Rice and products made from rice, like rice flour, Rice Krispies, rice
    cakes and rice noodles
Fruit, except citrus fruit
Salad
Vegetables, except potatoes

Eggs
Fish, including shellfish
Meat and poultry
Vegetable oils

## *Variations*

The following variations apply and must be strictly adhered to if you suffer from these symptoms:

### For constipation

No ordinary tea or decaffeinated tea whatsoever.
Two cups of coffee a day are allowed.
Concentrate on eating extra fruit, vegetables and salad.
Take at least two tablespoons of golden linseeds (Linusit Gold) daily with your cereal.
Take extra supplements of magnesium, preferably in the form of amino acid chelate (see page 248). You will need to take between 250 and 750mg per day, ideally last thing at night.

### For diarrhoea

No coffee whatsoever.
Two cups of tea are allowed.
No heavy spices.
No peppers or chilli.
Limited quantities of fruit, vegetables and salad, preferably eaten as small portions, little and often, rather than as part of a large meal.

### For wind

No foods containing sulphur.
No beans, onions or peppers.
None of the *Brassica* family, including cabbage, Brussels sprouts, broccoli.
Pay particular attention to avoiding yeast-based foods.
Try to avoid adding any sugar to your diet.

# The experiment – what it involves and how to prepare for it

The diet is broken down into several sections for good scientific reasons, and the rules should be followed throughout. It is extremely important that you consume only the foods and drinks that are allowed at the appropriate time. If you introduce foods that are not allowed in any section of the diet, you will lose the beneficial effects, and will probably have to start again, or at least go back to the basic two weeks for a few days, until your symptoms have calmed down.

There are eight Phases of the diet taking a total of ten weeks. You should follow each Phase in the sequence suggested.

Phase 1  Basic two weeks
Phase 2  Potato and corn week
Phase 3  Citrus week
Phase 4  Dairy products week
Phase 5  Yeast week
Phase 6  Oats, barley and rye week
Phase 7  White flour week
Phase 8  Wholewheat week

## Daily records

Your daily records will enable you to detect the cause of any reaction you may experience during each stage of the experiment. You will need to keep your symptom chart up to date every day. Probably the best time to complete it would be last thing at night, before you go to bed. You should also keep a record of the amount of exercise and relaxation you do each day.

## What to expect when you begin Phase 1

During the first week, it is quite common to suffer withdrawal symptoms to foods and drinks that have previously been part of your diet.

These can take the form of headaches, feelings of anxiety, tremor and shakes, fatigue, depression and even muscle weakness. Usually these pass within a few days, and are followed by an increased sense of well-being.

It is important to reach the stage when you experience an increased sense of well-being on Phase 1. It may well be, especially if you suffer with severe constipation, that you will need to be on this Phase for three weeks, instead of two, and in some rare cases for even four weeks. Do not be afraid to do an extra week if you are unsure. It will undoubtedly pay dividends in the long term, and will make it easier to tell if reactions are taking place.

## How to tell if you are experiencing a reaction

Unfortunately, reactions come in all shapes and sizes, and it is not simply a matter of us saying you will get a red spot over your left eye! In some cases, if you are unfortunate, the reaction will come on quite quickly after eating what for you is a trigger food. Sometimes the reaction can be almost immediate, and can cause sudden abdominal pain or bloating with lots of wind. These rapid reactions are very easy to detect, because you can't fail to miss them. The second type of reaction, the 'creeping' reaction, is far more difficult to detect, as it comes on gradually, sometimes over a period of a few weeks. The symptoms return so gradually that you hardly even notice it's happening, and it is not until you look back that you realize that you have experienced a reaction to something. This is where your daily records become worth their weight in gold. You will be able to refer back to them to see where precisely the loss of well-being or the gut symptoms themselves began to recur.

## What to do if you experience a reaction

As soon as you are sure that a reaction to a food or drink has occurred, you should stop eating or drinking the offending foods or drinks. It is advisable to go back to Phase 1 each time this happens, until you feel that things have settled down again. This varies from person to person and can take anything from a few days to a whole week.

You will need to keep careful notes on your daily chart about the food or drink that you suspect may be aggravating your symptoms. Once a food or drink has been placed on this list, you should continue to avoid it for the duration of the experiment. At the end of the book you will find instructions about re-introducing offending foods and drinks in the long term.

# Preparing for the experiment

Ideally, you should start this experiment when you are able to take a few days off, or perhaps over a long weekend. You will certainly need to be free of pressing commitments, as you may feel like crawling into bed and hiding away from the world.

If you are female, and of childbearing age, start after your period, rather than when you are premenstrual.

First, you need to read through Phase 1, and the notes you have made, and from these put a shopping list together. If you are going to stick to the diet rigidly, you must make sure that you have a good supply of the foods and drinks you can eat. If you have the time and enjoy cooking, then you may prefer to prepare some food in advance. Then, if you do feel low for the first few days, you won't have to put in much effort.

If you are out at work at lunchtime, you will need to think about what you can take along with you for lunch and do the necessary shopping in advance. See the section on Fast options at the beginning of each Phase.

Phase 1, the first two weeks, is obviously the most restricted Phase of the diet, You will undoubtedly find yourself eating a lot of rice and rice-based products, in order to feel even vaguely satisfied. Once you arrive at Phase 2, if you can manage to add potatoes and corn back into your diet without any problems, you will find it a lot easier to cope with.

You may find that you lose a little weight during the course of the experiment. If you are currently overweight, then this will be welcome news. However, if you are underweight, you must make sure that you concentrate on eating regularly, especially foods that contain lots of calories, like nuts, seeds, oily salad dressings, and bananas, assuming you can tolerate these well.

Try to enjoy the diet, even though you are bound to miss some of the forbidden foods and drinks that you really like. Being free from your severe symptoms will make up for it in the long run, so keep this in the forefront of your mind during each and every Phase.

As long as your diet is varied, interesting and enjoyable, you will not find it difficult to stick to. Most patients agree that they would willingly trade a few foods and drinks for their health.

We wish you well on your way, and hope that the experiment will provide you with the key to health as it has done for many others before you.

## Personal Therapy Plan

It is essential that you keep a record of your main symptoms at the beginning and end of the experiment. Note down the dates when you start the diet and the different sections of it, the type of supplements or laxatives that you decide to take, any additional modifications to the diet that you may need to make and any changes in your weight.

The purpose is to provide you with a written record of how you were and are, what you have done (and when), what you are doing now, and how you got on. To complete the first part of this Plan, you will have to have carefully decided what you are going to do so that you stick to it. Then as you progress, you complete the second part of the Plan which will record how you are getting on with it; in this way you will not get lost.

When you finish the Plan, you should have some firm conclusions or at least a very good idea of the dietary and other factors that can influence your IBS. Armed with this information you can take control of your future.

# Therapy Plan Chart

## *Symptoms at start of diet plan*

|  | NONE | MILD | MODERATE | SEVERE |
|---|---|---|---|---|
| 1 ABDOMINAL PAIN | | | | ✓ |
| 2 ABDOMINAL BLOATING | | ✓ – ✓ | | |
| 3 WIND DOWNWARDS | | ✓ | | |
| 4 NAUSEA | ✓ | | | |
| 5 URGENT NEED TO GO TO THE TOILET | | ✓ | | |
| 6 PAIN WHEN NEEDING TO GO TO THE TOILET | ✓ | | | |

7 HOW MANY TIMES DO YOU GO TO THE TOILET IN THE AVERAGE WEEK?
1–2 (SEVERE CONSTIPATION) _____
3–5 (CONSTIPATION) ___✓___ ?
6–13 (NORMAL FREQUENCY) _____
14–21 (SLIGHT DIARRHOEA) _____
22 OR MORE (DIARRHOEA) _____

8 WHAT DESCRIPTION BEST DESCRIBES THE APPEARANCE OF YOUR STOOLS?
PELLETY _____
THIN STRINGY SAUSAGES ___✓___
FAT SAUSAGES BUT HARD AND DRY _____
FAT SOFT SAUSAGES ___✓___
SLIGHTLY LOOSE BUT STILL STICKING TOGETHER _____
LOOSE, STILL JUST FORMED BUT NOT WATERY _____
WATERY AND NOT FORMED AT ALL _____

9 DO YOUR STOOLS VARY MUCH FROM ONE TYPE TO ANOTHER? ___✓___

## *Planning your therapy*

WHEN DO YOU INTEND TO START THE TEN-WEEK DIETARY PLAN? ___~~____~~___

ARE YOU ABLE TO EAT THREE REGULAR MEALS EACH DAY? ___✓___

DO YOU NEED TO MAKE ANY CHANGES TO YOUR ROUTINE TO ACHIEVE THIS? ___✗___

HOW OFTEN DO YOU REALISTICALLY THINK
THAT YOU WIL BE ABLE TO EXERCISE EACH WEEK? _3x_
WHAT WILL YOU DO? _CYCLE?/SWIM/AEROBIC_

DO YOU NEED PERIODS OF DAILY RELAXATION
TO HELP WITH STRESS-INDUCED BOWEL SYMPTOMS? _×_
IF YES, HOW MANY TIMES A DAY AND AT WHAT TIMES? _?_

## *Planning your supplements*

Do you need to take any of the following laxatives, medicines or supplements? Think carefully about each one and refer back to the relevant part of the book if in doubt.

|  |  | YES | NO |
|---|---|---|---|
| 1 | LINSEEDS: 1–2 TABLESPOONS PER DAY | ✓ | |
| 2 | BULK LAXATIVE e.g. ISOGEL/FYBOGEL | ✓ | |
| 3 | OTHER LAXATIVE PREPARATION e.g. FROM YOUR DOCTOR | | |
| 4 | SENNA ONLY TAKEN ONCE OR TWICE A WEEK | | |
| 5 | MAGNESIUM TABLETS: 250–500mg MAGNESIUM PER DAY | | |
| 6 | SUPPLEMENTS OF STRONG VITAMIN B COMPLEX: 50–100mg A DAY | | |
| 7 | SUPPLEMENTS FOR PREMENSTRUAL SYNDROME | | |
| 8 | SUPPLEMENTS FOR PREMENSTRUAL BREAST TENDERNESS | ✓ | |
| 9 | DO YOU NEED TO SPEAK TO YOUR DOCTOR ABOUT YOUR CURRENT DRUG THERAPY IN CASE THIS IS AGGRAVATING YOUR BOWEL SYMPTOMS? | | |

*(handwritten: EPO bracketing items 7 and 8)*

## *Planning your diet*

In addition to the diet that follows this chapter, there may be some additional dietary changes to make. Here are some questions about these possibilities to help you decide.

|  | YES | NO |
|---|---|---|
| DO YOU NEED TO LOSE WEIGHT? | | ✓ |

If yes, you will need to avoid calorie-rich foods.

DO YOU NEED TO AVOID THE ADDITIONAL FOODS
THAT CAN BE ASSOCIATED WITH EXCESSIVE WIND?       ____ _✓_
Consider avoiding foods that are hard to digest.

DO YOU PRODUCE OFFENSIVE SMELLING WIND?       _✓_ ____
Avoid foods which are high in sulphites.

ARE YOU KNOWN TO BE ALLERGIC OR
INTOLERANT TO ANY TYPES OF FOOD OR DRINK?       ____ _✓_
Avoid these foods.

DO YOU ALREADY FOLLOW A SPECIALIZED
DIET FROM YOUR DOCTOR OR FROM A HOSPITAL?       ____ ____
E.g. for diabetes, high cholesterol and kidney disease.
If yes, seek advice from your doctor or dietician.

## Symptoms at the end of the diet plan

|   | NONE | MILD | MODERATE | SEVERE |
|---|---|---|---|---|
| 1 ABDOMINAL PAIN | ____ | ____ | ____ | ____ |
| 2 ABDOMINAL BLOATING | ____ | ____ | ____ | ____ |
| 3 WIND DOWNWARDS | ____ | ____ | ____ | ____ |
| 4 NAUSEA | ____ | ____ | ____ | ____ |
| 5 URGENT NEED TO GO TO THE TOILET | ____ | ____ | ____ | ____ |
| 6 PAIN WHEN NEEDING TO GO TO THE TOILET | ____ | ____ | ____ | ____ |

7 HOW MANY TIMES DO YOU GO TO THE TOILET IN THE AVERAGE
   WEEK?
   1–2 (SEVERE CONSTIPATION) _____
   3–5 (CONSTIPATION) _____
   6–13 (NORMAL FREQUENCY) _____
   14–21 (SLIGHT DIARRHOEA) _____
   22 OR MORE (DIARRHOEA) _____

8 WHAT DESCRIPTION BEST DESCRIBES THE APPEARANCE OF YOUR
STOOLS?
PELLETY _____
THIN STRINGY SAUSAGES _____
FAT SAUSAGES BUT HARD AND DRY _____
FAT SOFT SAUSAGES _____
SLIGHTLY LOOSE BUT STILL STICKING TOGETHER _____
LOOSE, STILL JUST FORMED BUT NOT WATERY _____
WATERY AND NOT FORMED AT ALL _____

9 DO YOUR STOOLS VARY MUCH FROM ONE TYPE TO
ANOTHER? _____

# DAILY SYMPTOM CHART

| | Symptoms | Reaction | Exercise | Relaxation | Medication |
|---|---|---|---|---|---|
| Phase 1 | | | | | |
| Phase 2 | | | | | |
| Phase 3 | | | | | |
| Phase 4 | | | | | |

Phase 5

Phase 6

Phase 7

Phase 8

# REACTION DIARY

| | Safe foods/drinks | Uncertain foods/drinks | Foods/drinks to avoid |
|---|---|---|---|
| Phase 1 | | | |
| Phase 2 | | | |
| Phase 3 | | | |
| Phase 4 | | | |

Phase 5

Phase 6

Phase 7

Phase 8

# Phase 1
# the first two weeks

_____**Fast options**_____

## *Lunches*

Mackerel and salad
Pilchards and salad
Sardines and salad
Tuna and salad

Prawn and Rice Salad (page 117)
Rice salad with chicken
Rice salad with nuts

Avocado and salad

Chicken and salad
Ham and salad
Turkey and salad

Followed by fresh fruit or nuts or soya yoghurt and fruit.

## *Dinners*

Chicken with vegetables and rice
Lamb chops and vegetables
Steak and vegetables
Grilled plaice with vegetables and rice
Steamed salmon with vegetables and rice
Stir-fried vegetables and rice, with prawns, nuts or chicken
Tomato omelette with vegetables
Prawn and egg salad
Cold meat salad
Grilled fish with rice and salad

# Drinks and snacks

(These may be taken at any time during the ten-week plan, but use soya milk instead of cow's milk until the dairy week.)

## Hot drinks

Chicory
2 cups of coffee (if no diarrhoea)
Dandelion coffee (boiled root) or instant dandelion coffee (if not
    intolerant to lactose)
Rooibosch, Eleven O'clock tea (especially good for gut spasm)
Herbal teas, including fruit teas
2 cups of tea (if not constipated)

## Cold drinks

Avoid alcohol
Apple juice/Appletise
Bottled water (with or without gas)
Tonic water

# Snacks

Baked Apple (page 125) or pear
Coconut Rounds (page 125)
Fruit salad (without citrus fruit)
Fruit sorbet (see recipes, pages 126, 153 and 154)
Gooseberry Jelly
Non-citrus fruits
Rice cakes, with sugar-free jam or mashed banana or hazelnut or
    almond butter
Rice salad
Soya ice cream
Soya yoghurt

# Menus

## Day 1

### Breakfast

Rice Krispies, soya milk and chopped banana
Rice cakes *or* rice bread (toasted) with sugar-free jam

## Lunch

Canned sardines
Rice salad
Ginger and Carrot Salad (page 124)

## Dinner

Lamb and Apricot Pilaff (page 115)
Cauliflower
Carrots
Spinach

Baked Apple

## *Day 2*

## Breakfast

2 boiled eggs
Rice cakes *or* rice bread (toasted) with sugar-free jam

## Lunch

Fish Balls (page 118)
Green salad

## Dinner

Nut and Vegetable Loaf (page 121)
Green beans
Courgettes
Baked parsnips

Rhubarb and Ginger Mousse (page 127)

## *Day 3*

## Breakfast

Chopped apple and pear with soya yoghurt
Rice cakes *or* rice bread (toasted) with sugar-free jam

## Lunch

Sliced turkey breast
Endive fruit and nut salad
*or* white rice and watercress salad

## Dinner
Stuffed Mackerel (page 119)
Brussels sprouts
Carrots

Gooseberry Jelly

## *Day 4*

## Breakfast
2 poached eggs and 2 grilled rashers of bacon and tomato

## Lunch
Seafood Salad (page 117)

## Dinner
Chicken with Almonds (page 112)
Broccoli
Carrots
Swede

Blackcurrant Sorbet (page 126)

## *Day 5*

## Breakfast
Kedgeree (page 120)
Sliced peach

## Lunch

Nutty Quorn Risotto (page 120)
Fresh fruit

## Dinner
Lamb Casserole (page 116)
Cabbage
Carrots
Mange-touts

Baked pear

## Day 6

**Breakfast**

Rice Krispies with almonds, grapes and soya milk

**Lunch**

Salmon Scramble (page 119)
Mixed salad

**Dinner**

Beef Stir-fry with Apricots and Walnuts (page 114)
Boiled rice with courgettes and green beans

Coconut Rounds (page 125)

## Day 7

**Breakfast**

Soya yoghurt with chopped fruit and nuts
Rice cakes *or* rice bread (toasted) with sugar-free jam

**Lunch**

Canned tuna in brine
Courgette and Cauliflower Salad (page 124)
Rice and watercress salad

Fresh fruit

**Dinner**

Baked Chicken Burgers (page 112)
Cauliflower
Brussels sprouts
Peas

Fruit salad

## Day 8

**Breakfast**

2 egg omelette
2 grilled tomatoes
Rice cakes *or* rice bread (toasted) with sugar-free jam

## Lunch

Mackerel in tomato sauce
Mixed salad
Mini popadoms

## Dinner

Vegetable Loaf with Mustard Sauce (page 122)
Parsnips
Turnips
Swede

Melon Balls (page 124)

# *Day 9*

## Breakfast

Rice Krispies with chopped fruit and nuts and soya milk
Rice cakes *or* rice bread (toasted) with sugar-free jam

## Lunch

Lean ham
Apple and Nut Salad (page 123)
Green salad

## Dinner

Prawn and Vegetable Stir-fry (page 118)
Rice

Chopped fresh fruit and soya yoghurt

# *Day 10*

## Breakfast

2 scrambled eggs and grilled tomatoes with rice cakes or rice
bread (toasted)

## Lunch

Canned salmon
Beansprouts
Rice and watercress salad

## Dinner

Provençale Stew (page 113)
Cabbage
Mange-touts

Fruit Snow (page 126)

## *Day 11*

## Breakfast

Chopped fruit and nuts with soya yoghurt
Rice cakes *or* rice bread (toasted) with sugar-free jam

## Lunch

Sliced chicken
Root salad *or* mixed salad

## Dinner

Grilled plaice
Greens
Carrots
Parsnips

Baked Apple (page 125)

## *Day 12*

## Breakfast

Grilled bacon and tomatoes *or* rice bread (toasted) with sugar-free jam

## Lunch

Prawn and Rice Salad (page 117)

## Dinner

Spinach and Tomato Omelette (page 122)
Baked Nutty Onions (page 123)
Brussels sprouts

Coconut Rounds (page 125)

## *Day 13*

### Breakfast

2 poached eggs
Rice cakes *or* rice bread (toasted) with sugar-free jam

### Lunch

Canned tuna in brine
Egg and Cabbage Salad (page 124)
Grated carrot, sesame seeds and sesame oil dressing

### Dinner

Lamb and Aubergine Bake (page 115)
Boiled rice
Broccoli
Carrots

Rhubarb and Ginger Mousse (page 127)

## *Day 14*

### Breakfast

Rice Krispies with chopped fruit and nuts and soya milk

### Lunch

Chicken drumstick
Coleslaw
Courgette and Cauliflower Salad (page 124)

### Dinner

Salmon Steaks with Ginger (page 119)
Peas
Mixed salad

Gooseberry Jelly

## Recipes

(These recipes are suitable for all phases of the plan.)

### *Main courses*

### Baked Chicken Burgers

SERVES 4

450 g (1 lb) cooked chicken meat, minced or finely chopped
1 egg, beaten
1 garlic clove, crushed
1 tbsp finely chopped fresh parsley
2 tsp dried tarragon
freshly ground black pepper to taste
1 tbsp sunflower oil
1 onion, finely chopped

Mix together the chicken and egg in a mixing bowl. Add the garlic, parsley, tarragon and pepper, and mix well. Heat the oil in frying pan and gently fry the onion for 2-3 minutes. Add the onion to the chicken mixture and stir well. Form the mixture into round burger shapes and place on a greased baking sheet. Bake in a preheated oven at Gas Mark 4 (180°C, 350°F) for 15-20 minutes or until golden brown, turning half way through baking.

### Chicken with Almonds

SERVES 4-6

2 tbsp vegetable oil
1 × 2.25 kg (5 lb) chicken, cut into 8 serving pieces
1 large onion, finely chopped
2 garlic cloves, crushed (optional)
1 large green pepper, seeded and chopped
1 large red pepper, seeded and chopped
450 ml (¾ pint) chicken stock
1 pinch cayenne pepper
bouquet garni consisting of 4 parsley sprigs, 1 thyme spray and 1 bay leaf tied together
2 hard-boiled egg yolks
50 g (2 oz) ground almonds

Heat the oil in a large flameproof casserole dish over a moderate heat. Add the chicken pieces and brown gently on both sides. Remove the chicken and set aside.

Place the onion, garlic, green and red peppers in the casserole dish and cook, stirring occasionally, for 5-7 minutes or until the onion is soft but not brown. Add the chicken to the casserole along with the stock, cayenne pepper and bouquet garni. Bring the liquid to the boil, reduce the heat and simmer for 40 minutes or until the chicken is tender.

In a small bowl mash the egg yolks together with 3 tablespoons of the cooking liquid with a fork until the mixture forms a smooth paste. Add the ground almonds and combine the mixture thoroughly. Stir the paste into the casserole a little at a time and simmer for a further 10 minutes.

Remove the chicken pieces from the casserole and transfer to a warmed serving dish. Discard the bouquet garni and continue to boil the sauce, stirring occasionally, for 3-5 minutes until thickened slightly. Remove the casserole from the heat and pour the sauce over the chicken. Serve immediately.

## Provençale Stew

### SERVES 4

450 g (1 lb) stewing steak
25 g (1 oz) cornflour
freshly ground black pepper
2 tbsp corn oil
2 onions, sliced
1 clove garlic, crushed
2 carrots, sliced
600 ml (1 pint) beef stock
1 small red pepper, diced
1 small green pepper, diced

Trim the meat and cut it into cubes. Coat well with cornflour, seasoned with pepper. Heat the corn oil and gently fry the meat, onions, garlic and carrots. Add the beef stock and peppers, cover and simmer gently for 1-1¼ hours or until the meat is tender.

## Beef Stir-fry with Apricots and Walnuts

SERVES 4

6 fresh or dried apricots
350 g (12 oz) rump steak
2 tsp cornflour
4 tbsp water
4 tbsp orange juice
2 tsp groundnut (peanut) or vegetable oil
4 spring onions, cut diagonally into 2.5 cm (1 inch) pieces
1 tbsp wheat-free tamari
3 medium Chinese leaves, roughly chopped
50 g (2 oz) walnut pieces
freshly ground black pepper to taste

If using dried apricots, soak them in cold water for 1 hour, then drain and cut them into quarters. If using fresh apricots, stone them and cut them into quarters.

Remove any fat from the steak, wrap the meat in cling film and place it in the freezer for about 45 minutes or until nearly frozen.

Remove the meat from the freezer and cut it across the grain into very thin strips.

Blend the cornflour with 1 tbsp water, then add the rest of the water and the orange juice.

Heat the oil in a wok or frying pan. Add the meat and stir-fry for 3-4 minutes or until browned. Reduce the heat to moderate, add the onions, wheat-free tamari and Chinese leaves, and continue to stir-fry for a further minute.

Add the apricots and cornflour mixture to the pan and bring to the boil over a moderate to high heat, stirring constantly. After about 30 seconds, the mixture should become thick and glossy.

Remove the pan from the heat and stir in the walnuts. Season with pepper and serve immediately.

## Lamb and Apricot Pilaff

SERVES 4

30 ml (2 tbsp) sunflower oil
1 medium onion, thinly sliced
700 g (1½ lb) boned leg of lamb, cut into 2.5cm (1 inch) cubes
75 g (3 oz) dried apricots, soaked overnight, drained and halved
3 tbsp raisins
½ tsp ground cinnamon
freshly ground black pepper
900 ml (1½ pints) water
225 g (8 oz) long-grain rice, washed, soaked in cold water for 30 minutes and drained

Heat the oil in a frying pan, add the onion and cook for about 5 minutes, until translucent but not brown.

Add the lamb and cook, stirring and turning occasionally, for 5-8 minutes, or until it is lightly browned all over. Stir in the apricots, raisins, cinnamon and pepper.

Pour in 450 ml (6 fl oz) of the water and bring to the boil, stirring occasionally. Reduce the heat to low, cover the pan and simmer the meat for 1-1¼ hours, or until the meat is tender when pierced with the point of a sharp knife.

Cook the rice in the usual way, using the remaining water.

Preheat the oven to Gas Mark 4 (180°C, 350°F).

Place one-third of the rice in a medium ovenproof casserole. Cover with a layer of one-third of the meat mixture, then top with another one-third of the rice. Continue to make layers in this manner until all the ingredients have been used up, finishing with a layer of rice. Cover the casserole and bake for 50 minutes. Serve immediately.

## Lamb and Aubergine Bake

SERVES 2

250 g (9 oz) aubergine
2 tsp vegetable oil
1 small onion, chopped
1 clove garlic, finely chopped
15 g (½ oz) cooked brown rice
1 tbsp canned sweetcorn
200 g (7 oz) minced lamb
1 tbsp tomato purée

Preheat the oven to Gas Mark 5 (190°C, 375°F). Cut the aubergine in half lengthways. Lightly score inside each half with a sharp knife. Sprinkle with salt and leave for 20-30 minutes, then rinse thoroughly in cold water.

Remove and chop the white flesh, reserving the hollow halves.

Heat the oil, and gently fry the onion and garlic for 2-3 minutes. Add the white aubergine flesh and stir for 2 more minutes. Add the rice, sweetcorn, lamb and tomato purée to the pan. Season with pepper, and stir for 2-3 minutes to brown the meat.

Spoon this mixture into the aubergine halves, cover and bake for 20-25 minutes. Remove and serve immediately.

## Lamb Casserole

### SERVES 4

1 kg (2 lb) lamb neck chops, trimmed
4 tbsp seasoned corn flour
3 tbsp vegetable oil
750 g (1½ lb) potatoes, peeled and thinly sliced
1 large onion, chopped
2 large carrots, sliced
1 large leek, sliced
freshly ground black pepper
dried mixed herbs
450 ml (¾ pint) lamb stock

Preheat the oven to Gas Mark 4 (180°C, 350°F). Pat the chops dry and roll them in the seasoned flour. Heat the oil in a large saucepan, brown the lamb all over and set aside. Line the base of a large casserole dish with half of the sliced potatoes. Mix together the vegetables, seasoning and mixed herbs in a bowl. Arrange layers of the vegetables and lamb in the casserole dish beginning and ending with vegetables. Top with the rest of the potato slices.

Pour over the stock, cover with buttered foil and a tight-fitting lid. Cook in the oven for 1½-2 hours. Remove the lid and foil and grill for a few minutes to brown the top.

## Prawn and Rice Salad

### SERVES 4

350 g (12 oz) cold cooked basmati rice
1 stick celery, thinly sliced
100 g (4 oz) cooked peas
225 g (8 oz) peeled prawns
4 tbsp mayonnaise
grated rind of ½ lemon
freshly ground black pepper
pinch of paprika
8 lettuce leaves, washed
6 sprigs of dill to garnish

Place the rice, celery, peas and prawns (reserving a few for the garnish) in a large mixing bowl. Add the mayonnaise and lemon rind and toss gently until all the ingredients are coated. Season with black pepper and paprika. Line a salad bowl with the lettuce leaves and pile the salad into the centre. Garnish with the reserved prawns and dill.

## Seafood Salad

### SERVES 4

225 g (8 oz) squid, thinly sliced
450 g (1 lb) mussels, cooked
100 g (4 oz) peeled prawns
2 tomatoes, sliced
1 small onion, finely chopped
1 clove garlic, crushed
1 tbsp white wine vinegar
1 tbsp chopped fresh parsley
1 tbsp fresh lemon juice
2 tbsp white wine
freshly ground black pepper to taste

Cook the squid in a pan of boiling water for 2-3 minutes. Remove and leave to drain.

Mix together the squid and all the remaining ingredients and chill in the refrigerator before serving.

## Prawn and Vegetable Stir-fry

### SERVES 4

3 tbsp vegetable oil
100 g (4 oz) broccoli, divided into florets
100 g (4 oz) carrots, cut into small matchstick size pieces
100 g (4 oz) leeks, thinly sliced
225 g (8 oz) peeled prawns
50 g (2 oz) courgettes, thinly sliced
100 g (4 oz) Chinese leaves, roughly chopped
1 apple, cored and diced
1 tbsp grated ginger
100 g (4 oz) onions, chopped
1 tbsp lemon juice

Heat the oil in a wok or large frying-pan. Add the broccoli, carrots and leeks and cook for 3 minutes. Add the prawns, courgettes, Chinese leaves, apple, ginger, onions and lemon juice and cook for a further 2 minutes. Serve immediately.

## Fish Balls

### MAKES 30-34 FISH BALLS

450 g (1 lb) skinned and filleted white fish
1 egg white
2 tsp cornflour
2 tsp vegetable oil
2 tbsp finely chopped fresh coriander
freshly ground black pepper to taste
900 ml (1½ pints) fish stock

Place the fish in a blender and purée until smooth. Add the egg white, cornflour, oil, coriander and pepper. Blend again until thoroughly combined, then turn into a bowl.

Divide the mixture into 30-34 small balls. Refrigerate for 25-30 minutes.

Place the fish stock in a large saucepan and bring to the boil. Drop the fish balls into the stock and simmer gently for 5-6 minutes. Serve hot with vegetables and a sauce, or cold with salad.

Alternatively, instead of cooking in stock the fish balls can be stir-fried for 4-5 minutes in oil flavoured with garlic.

## Stuffed Mackerel

SERVES 2

1 orange
1 apple, grated
1 tbsp finely chopped fresh parsley
1 medium onion, finely chopped
2 tbsp cooked brown rice
2 × 140 g (5 oz) fresh mackerel, gutted
1 tsp dried rosemary or 4 sprigs fresh rosemary

Preheat the oven to Gas Mark 6 (200°C, 400°F).

Grate the peel of the orange and chop the flesh into small pieces, discarding the pips.

Mix the grated orange peel and flesh with the apple, parsley, onion and rice.

Divide the mixture into 2 and use to stuff the mackerel loosely. Place the rosemary in each fish. Wrap the fish in foil and bake in the oven for about 40 minutes.

## Salmon Steaks with Ginger

SERVES 2

2 salmon steaks
2 tbsp lemon juice
2.5 cm (1 inch) square of fresh root ginger, peeled and finely chopped
freshly ground black pepper to taste

Preheat the oven to Gas Mark 4 (180°C, 350°F).

Place each salmon steak on a large piece of foil. Add 1 tablespoon of lemon juice and half the chopped ginger to each steak. Season with a little black pepper. Wrap the steaks individually in foil to make two parcels, and bake in the oven for 20 minutes. Serve hot with vegetables, or cold with salad.

## Salmon Scramble

SERVES 2

3 eggs
1 tbsp skimmed milk
2 tsp chopped dill
freshly ground black pepper
75 g (3 oz) canned salmon

Whisk the eggs and milk and stir in the dill and freshly ground black pepper. Cook gently in a non-stick pan, stirring constantly, for 4-5 minutes until firm. Mix in the salmon, and serve.

## ✓ Kedgeree
### SERVES 2

175 g (6 oz) unsmoked haddock, filleted and skinned
75 g (3 oz) brown rice
1 hard-boiled egg, chopped
½ green pepper, seeded and chopped
2 tbsp natural yoghurt
1 small onion, finely chopped
1 sprig parsley, chopped
freshly ground black pepper to taste
2 slices lemon to garnish

Cover the fish with water in a shallow pan. Heat gently and poach for about 8-10 minutes. Remove the fish, and flake.

Boil the rice in the poaching water left in the pan according to the instructions on the rice packet. You may need to add extra water.

Drain the rice, stir in the fish, egg, green pepper, yoghurt, onion and parsley, and mix well. Heat gently, stirring all the time. Season with pepper, and serve garnished with the lemon slices.

## Nutty Quorn Risotto
### SERVES 4

225 g (8 oz) brown rice
1 tbsp sunflower oil
1 medium onion, sliced
1 clove garlic, crushed
1 red pepper, seeded and sliced
1 green pepper, seeded and sliced
50 g (2 oz) green beans
100 g (4 oz) carrots, cut into matchsticks
100 g (4 oz) courgettes, thinly sliced
100 g (4 oz) broccoli, broken into florets and stalk sliced
225 g (8 oz) Quorn
1 small seedless orange with skin removed, broken into segments
1 tbsp flaked almonds
1 tbsp fresh chopped parsley

Cook the rice as directed on the packet and put to one side.

Heat the oil in a large frying pan and add the onion, garlic, red and green peppers and gently fry for 2-3 minutes.

Steam the beans, carrots, courgettes and broccoli over a pan of boiling water for 5 minutes (alternatively miss the steaming if you like your vegetables crunchy). Place in the frying pan with the onion, garlic and peppers. Add the Quorn, orange, flaked almonds, parsley and rice, and heat through until all the ingredients are hot. Serve immediately.

## Nut and Vegetable Loaf

### SERVES 4-6

2 tsp sunflower oil
1 small onion, chopped
1 small carrot, chopped
1 stick celery, chopped
1 tbsp tomato purée
225 g (8 oz) tomatoes, skinned and chopped
2 eggs
1 tbsp freshly chopped parsley
freshly ground black pepper to taste
225 g (8 oz) mixed nuts, finely chopped or minced
onion rings and parsley sprigs to garnish

Preheat the oven to Gas Mark 7 (220°C, 425°F).

Heat the oil in pan, add the onion, carrot and celery and cook until softened. Add the tomato purée and tomatoes and cook for 5 minutes.

Place the eggs, parsley and pepper in a mixing bowl and beat well. Stir in the nuts and vegetable mixture. Transfer to a lightly greased 900 ml (1½ pint) ovenproof dish and bake for 30-35 minutes. Turn out on to a plate and garnish with the onion rings and parsley sprigs. Serve hot with vegetables and a sauce, or cold with salad.

## Vegetable Loaf with Mustard Sauce

SERVES 4

225 g (8 oz) carrot, coarsely grated
175 g (6 oz) cooked white or brown rice
100 g (4 oz) potato, peeled and grated
100 g (4 oz) onion, finely chopped
100 g (4 oz) celery, chopped
75 g (3 oz) green pepper, chopped
1 tsp paprika
2 medium eggs, beaten

*Sauce*
25 g (1 oz) polyunsaturated margarine
25 g (1 oz) potato or rice flour
300 ml (½ pint) skimmed milk
made from non-dairy milk powder
1½ tsp mustard

Line a 13 × 20 cm (5 × 8 inch) loaf tin with foil.

Combine all the vegetable ingredients and the paprika and eggs in a bowl, then press the mixture into the loaf tin. Bake in a preheated oven at Gas Mark 4 (180°C, 350°F) for 50 minutes. Remove from the oven and leave to stand while making the sauce.

To make the sauce, melt the margarine in a saucepan, stir in the flour and cook for 1-2 minutes, stirring constantly. Slowly add the milk, again stirring all the time over a low heat until the sauce thickens. Stir in the mustard.

Turn the vegetable loaf out on to a plate. Slice, and serve with the sauce.

## Spinach and Tomato Omelette

SERVES 1

2 eggs
freshly ground black pepper
50 g (2 oz) fresh spinach (cooked in a little boiling water for 3-4 minutes and drained)
2 medium tomatoes, sliced

Beat the eggs and mix with the pepper. Pour into a hot frying pan and leave to set for ½ minute.

Add the spinach and tomatoes and leave for about a minute until heated through. Fold in half and serve.

## *Side dishes*

### Baked Nutty Onions

SERVES 4

300 g (10 oz) onions, sliced
1 bay leaf
300 ml (½ pint) skimmed milk
25 g (1 oz) sunflower margarine
25 g (1 oz) cornflour
freshly ground black pepper to taste
1 tsp ground nutmeg
150 g (5 oz) unsalted peanuts, finely chopped
2 tomatoes, halved and grilled

Preheat the oven to Gas Mark 5 (190°C, 375°F). Place the onion, bay leaf and milk in a saucepan and bring to the boil. Cover, and simmer for 10 minutes. Strain the milk into a jug, discard the bay leaf and place the onions in a greased ovenproof dish.

Melt the margarine in a small pan. When foaming, stir in the cornflour and cook for 1 minute. Gradually add the milk, stirring continuously. Cook until thick and smooth. Add the pepper and nutmeg to taste. Pour the sauce over the onions and sprinkle evenly with the nuts. Bake for 20-30 minutes. Reduce the heat if the nuts are browning too quickly. Garnish with the grilled tomatoes before serving.

### Apple and Nut Salad

SERVES 4

4 red apples, wiped
lemon juice, to coat
½ cucumber, thickly sliced
6 sticks celery, chopped
1 bunch spring onions, sliced
75 g (3 oz) natural peanuts

Core and roughly chop the apples and dip them in the lemon juice to prevent discolouration. Cut the cucumber slices into quarters.

Mix all the ingredients together and toss in a dressing of your choice.

## Courgette and Cauliflower Salad

SERVES 4

75 g (3 oz) courgettes, thinly sliced
225 g (8 oz) cauliflower, cut into small florets
100 g (4 oz) red pepper, seeded and chopped
1 apple, chopped
1 tsp freshly chopped fennel, to garnish

Mix the courgettes, cauliflower, red pepper and apple together.
Serve garnished with the fennel.

## Egg and Cabbage Salad

SERVES 4

½ cabbage, finely grated
2 hard-boiled eggs, finely chopped
2 tbsp pine nuts
3 tbsp mayonnaise
curry powder to taste

Mix all the ingredients together.

## Ginger and Carrot Salad

SERVES 4

175 g (6oz) carrots, grated
2 medium apples, grated
1 tsp ground ginger
1 stick celery, chopped

Mix all the ingredients together.

# *Desserts*

## Melon Balls

SERVES 4

2 ripe honeydew melons, halved and seeded
½ tsp ground ginger

*To decorate*
mint sprigs
½ tbsp caster sugar

Remove as much of the melon flesh as you can using a melon baller or teaspoon. Catch the juices in a dish. Scoop out what is left of the melon flesh and purée in a blender. Combine with the melon balls and stir in the ginger. Cover with cling film and chill.

To serve, place the melon mixture in individual bowls and sprinkle with the caster sugar to taste. Garnish with mint sprigs.

## Coconut Rounds

MAKES 20 ROUNDS

2 egg whites
75 g (3 oz) desiccated coconut
25 g (1 oz) ground almonds
100 g (4 oz) caster sugar
10 glacé cherries, halved

Preheat the oven to Gas Mark 3 (160°C, 325°F) 10 minutes before cooking. Line a large baking sheet with baking parchment.

Whisk the egg whites until stiff and carefully fold in the coconut, almonds and sugar. Spoon 20 rounds of the mixture on to a baking sheet 5 cm (2 inches) apart. Place a cherry half on top of each. Bake for 20-25 minutes or until golden brown. Allow to cool before serving.

## Baked Apples

SERVES 4

4 cooking apples
1 tbsp honey or sugar-free jam

*For the stuffing*
50 g (2 oz) raisins or 25 g (1 oz) dates
brown sugar or honey to taste

Preheat the oven to Gas Mark 6 (200°C, 400°F). Wash and core the apples. Slit the skin of each in a horizontal ring around the middle. Stuff with your chosen filling mixed with brown sugar or honey. Add 2 cm (¼ inch) water and 1 tablespoon of honey to a baking dish. Bake until the fruit is tender – probably about 45 minutes but it depends on the size of the apples. Serve hot or cold.

## Blackcurrant Sorbet

SERVES 4-6

300 ml (½ pint) water
100 g (4 oz) granulated sugar
juice of half a lemon
450 g (1 lb) fresh or frozen blackcurrants
2 egg whites

Put the water and sugar in a heavy-based saucepan and heat gently until the sugar has dissolved. Bring to the boil, then simmer for 5 minutes or until syrupy. Remove from the heat, stir in the lemon juice and leave to cool.

Put the blackcurrants in a heavy-based saucepan and heat gently for 5-10 minutes or until the blackcurrants are soft and the juices run. Remove from the heat and press the blackcurrants through a sieve. Leave to cool.

Combine the syrup and blackcurrant purée. Pour the mixture into a freezer container, and chill in the refrigerator for at least 30 minutes.

Transfer the blackcurrant mixture to the freezer and freeze for 1-2 hours or until slushy.

Whisk the egg whites until stiff. Remove the blackcurrant mixture from the freezer and turn it out into a bowl. Beat thoroughly, then fold in the egg whites until evenly blended.

Return the sorbet mixture to the container, cover and freeze for at least 2 hours or until firm. (The sorbet can be stored in the freezer for up to 2 months.) Before serving, stand the sorbet at room temperature for 10-20 minutes to soften slightly. Scoop into individual bowls.

## Fruit Snow

SERVES 2

200 g (7 oz) dessert apples, peeled, cored and thinly sliced
grated rind of 1 orange
2 tbsp water
white of 1 large egg, beaten until stiff
2 slices orange to garnish

Place the apples, water and orange rind in a saucepan. Cover and cook gently, stirring occasionally until the apples are soft. Rub the apples through a sieve and leave to cool. Fold in the egg white, and chill before serving. Serve garnished with the orange slices.

## Rhubarb and Ginger Mousse

SERVES 4

450 g (1 lb) rhubarb
3 tbsp clear honey
juice and grated rind of half an orange
¼ tsp ground ginger
2 tbsp water
2 tsp powdered gelatine
2 egg whites

Trim the rhubarb and chop into 2.5 cm (1 inch) pieces. Place in a saucepan with the honey, orange juice, rind and the ginger and simmer gently until the fruit is soft. Place the water in a small heatproof bowl and sprinkle in the gelatine. Stand the bowl in a saucepan of hot water. Stir until the gelatine has dissolved. Add the gelatine mixture to the rhubarb mixture and beat until smooth. Leave to cool until half-set.

Whisk the egg whites until stiff and fold them lightly into the half-set rhubarb mixture. Spoon into four dessert glasses and chill until set.

# 18

# Phase 2
# potato and corn week

## Fast options

### Lunches

Mackerel and salad
Pilchards and salad
Sardines and salad
Tuna and salad

Prawn and Rice Salad (page 117)
Rice salad with chicken
Rice salad with nuts

Avocado and salad

Chicken and salad
Ham and salad
Turkey and salad

Jacket potato with fillings (baked beans, tuna and sweetcorn, prawns and celery)

Corn on the cob

### Dinner

Chicken with vegetables and rice
Lamb chops and vegetables
Steak and vegetables
Grilled plaice with vegetables and rice
Steamed salmon with vegetables and rice
Stir-fried vegetables and rice with prawns, nuts or chicken
Tomato omelette with vegetables
Prawn and egg salad
Cold meat salad
Grilled fish with rice and salad

Chips
Corn on the cob
Jacket potato
Mashed potato
Roast potatoes
Sweetcorn

## *Drinks and snacks*

(Use soya milk instead of cow's milk until dairy week.)

### Hot drinks

Chicory
2 cups of coffee (if no diarrhoea)
Dandelion coffee (boiled root) or instant dandelion coffee (if not
    intolerant to lactose)
Rooibosch, Eleven O'clock tea (especially good for gut spasm)
Herbal teas, including fruit teas
2 cups of tea (if not constipated)

### Cold drinks

Avoid alcohol
Apple juice/Appletise
Bottled water (with or without gas)
Tonic water

### Snacks

Baked Apple (page 125) or pear
Chips (if you are thin)
Coconut Rounds (page 125)
Corn crispbreads
Corn wafers/Nachips (corn chips)
Fruit salad (without citrus fruit)
Fruit sorbet (see recipes, pages 126; 153 and 154)
Glutano crackers
Gooseberry Jelly
Home-made bread with rice and potato flour
Low-fat plain potato crisps (in moderation)
Non-citrus fruits
Plain popcorn
Rice cakes, with sugar-free jam or mashed banana or hazelnut or
    almond butter
Rice salad
Soya ice cream
Soya yoghurt
Tacos

Although at this stage you will be following a restricted diet there are many alternatives available that you should be aware of. Some of these can be made by home baking, and other commercial products can be found in health-food shops or can be ordered by your pharmacist.

Before looking at the menu plan for Phase 2 you might like to consider some of the alternatives to incorporate into your diet at this stage.

# The gluten-free diet

Foods containing gluten are most commonly the grains wheat, oats, barley and rye. While people who suffer from coeliac disease know that they must avoid gluten, according to recent research there are many pre-coeliacs or gluten-sensitive individuals suffering from IBS who also would do well to avoid gluten.

## *Food allowances and cooking instructions*

Avoiding foods that contain gluten is not necessarily as easy as it sounds, for wheat, in particular, is used as a thickening agent in the form of modified starch in many types of food, ranging from yoghurts to sauces. In order to avoid gluten completely you will need to arm yourself with alternatives and to read food labels carefully before making purchases. There are plenty of alternatives; it is just a question of knowing what to look for.

## *Bread*

There are now many alternatives to ordinary bread, some of which can be purchased and others which you need to bake yourself. Both pharmacies and health-food shops usually have some stocks of the alternative grain products; in our experience pharmacies are usually the most reasonably priced. Behind pharmacy counters you will usually find a stock of products kept for people with gluten allergy. Ask the pharmacist for help as they sometimes have to order products on request.

Look out for some of the following products:

- 'Ener G' white or brown rice bread (which toasts nicely)
- 'Glutafin' wheat-free bread, rolls and crackers

- 'Glutano' crackers, part-baked and corn wafers are all very acceptable
- Rice cakes
- 'Orgran' Corn Crispbreads

It is possible to make something that resembles bread using a combination of rice, corn, potato or gram flour (see Potato and Rice Bread recipe, page 141).

## Pasta

Although you will need to avoid the pasta made with wheat there are many reasonable alternatives you can try. Most of these are available from health-food shops, Chinese supermarkets or pharmacies.

Pastariso make brown rice spaghetti, which is very acceptable when slightly undercooked. They also do a range of other pastas. Although some health-food shops do stock it, it is easier to order it from a pharmacy.

Glutafin have a range of pasta which is sometimes available in health-food shops and again can be ordered from chemists.

Rice noodles are available in a wide variety from Chinese supermarkets. There are wide, flat rice noodles that resemble tagliatelle, spaghetti-like noodles, and the very skinny variety that only need soaking in a covered pan in boiling water for a few minutes. You will probably find that these are cheaper than the alternative pastas available from health-food shops and chemists.

## Breakfast cereal

Any rice or corn cereals will be fine, even ordinary Rice Krispies and cornflakes from supermarkets. Add some chopped fruit and some crumbled nuts, perhaps a few seeds and a little dried fruit to your cereal to make it a bit more wholesome, or make a muesli using nuts, seeds, rice, corn and dried fruit. There are some alternative mueslis available, but they are usually very expensive for only a small packet.

## Home-made cakes

If you enjoy baking there are plenty of very acceptable biscuits, cakes, pastries, sponges and pancakes you can make using alternative flours. If you have never used any of the alternative flours before it may take you a little time to find consistency that you like.

**Sponges**   Brown rice flour is probably the best for making a sponge. Make it up to the weight given in the recipe by mixing it with a little ground almonds and a raising agent (cream of tartar and bicarbonate of soda – see below).

**Raising agents**   As baking powder contains wheat, you will need to use an alternative. Either use a combination of one part bicarbonate of soda to two parts of cream of tartar, or use Glutafin wheat-free baking powder.

## Savoury pancakes

These are best made with a combination of brown rice flour, or ground rice and cornflour, purchased from a health-food shop or Chinese supermarket. Use half cornflour and half rice flour to replace the normal quantity of flour in the ordinary pancake recipe.

## Breadcrumbs or batter

A crisp coating for fish or meat can be made with maize meal, which can be found in health-food shops. Coat the fish or meat with maize meal then with beaten egg and once again with maize meal. You can then bake, grill or even fry the food which should emerge with a crispy coat.

## Biscuits

There is a variety of biscuits that you can make using brown rice flour, or ground rice and ground nuts or coconut. If you make plain biscuits you can flavour them with lemon or ginger. Recipes for almond macaroons and coconut biscuits are very acceptable and at the same time more nutritious than the average biscuit, as they are full of eggs and nuts. It is a good idea to make some and keep them in the freezer so that you can take a few out when you really feel you need something sweet to eat.

There are many other flours that you can use in your cooking. Gram flour made from chickpeas, potato flour, soya flour, tapioca flour and millet flour are all good examples. Glutafin makes flour mixes for bread, pastry and cakes as does Tru Free, and these are available in some health-food shops.

## *Shop-bought cakes and biscuits*

Acceptable cakes and biscuits can now be purchased in health-food shops and ordered from most chemists.

Both Glutafin and Glutano have a range of biscuits including digestives, and Rite Diet have a range of biscuits and cakes. The coconut biscuits are the least sweet, and the banana or lemon cakes are worth trying too.

## *Snacks*

It is nice to have something to crunch on when you are avoiding wheat. There are lots of corn products available, but do remember to read the labels, as some contain wheat. Try corn crisps and wafers and look in the Mexican section of the supermarket. Also, poppadoms are fine, and little mini spiced poppadoms are delicious to nibble on or dip.

# Menus

## *Day 1*

### Breakfast

Chopped fruit and nuts with soya yoghurt
Rice cakes *or* rice (bread) toasted

### Lunch

Mackerel in tomato sauce
Jacket potato with butter
Green salad

### Dinner

Roast chicken
Roast potatoes
Cabbage
Carrots

Blackcurrant Sorbet (page 126)

## *Day 2*

### Breakfast

Rice Krispies with chopped fruit and nuts
Soya milk

### Lunch

Root Veggie Bake (page 140)
Mixed salad

### Dinner

Chicken, Spinach and Sweetcorn Soup (page 138)
Grilled lamb chops
Chips
Peas
Green beans

Baked pears

## *Day 3*

**Breakfast**
Scrambled egg and tomato *or* rice bread (toasted)

**Lunch**
Sliced turkey
Potato salad
Coleslaw

**Dinner**
Broccoli and Sweetcorn Stuffed Plaice (page 139)
Mashed potatoes
Carrots

Fruit salad

## *Day 4*

**Breakfast**
Cornflakes
Chopped fruit and nuts and soya milk
Rice cakes *or* rice bread (toasted) with sugar-free jam

**Lunch**
Fish Balls (page 118)
Mixed salad
Coleslaw
Nachips (corn chips)

**Dinner**
Nut and Vegetable Loaf (page 121)
Roast potatoes
Green beans

Melon Balls (page 124)

## *Day 5*

**Breakfast**
Cornflakes
Chopped fruit and nuts and soya milk
Rice cakes *or* rice bread (toasted) with sugar-free jam

## Lunch

Canned tuna in brine
Courgette and Cauliflower Salad (page 124)
Nachips (corn chips)

## Dinner

Liver and Sweetcorn (page 139)
Mange-touts
Duchesse potatoes
Carrots

Baked Apple (page 125)

# *Day 6*

## Breakfast

Cornflakes
Chopped fruit and nuts and soya milk
Rice cakes *or* rice bread (toasted) with sugar-free jam

## Lunch

Corn on the cob
Jacket potato
Green salad
Nachips (corn chips)

## Dinner

Chicken and Sweetcorn Risotto (page 138)
Green beans
Courgettes

Fruit Snow (page 126)

# *Day 7*

## Breakfast

Cornflakes
Chopped fruit and nuts and soya milk
Rice cakes *or* rice bread (toasted) with sugar-free jam

## Lunch

Sliced chicken
Coleslaw
Beansprout salad
Nachips (corn chips)

## Dinner

Leek and Potato Soup (page 137)
Corn Pasta with Mince and Spinach (page 140)

Coconut Rounds (page 125)

## Recipes

### *Soups*

### Leek and Potato Soup

SERVES 4

1 tbsp sunflower oil
2 carrots, peeled and sliced
2 leeks, trimmed, washed and sliced
1 large potato, peeled and sliced
freshly ground black pepper
450 ml (¾ pint) vegetable stock
150 ml (¼ pint) soya milk
4 small sprigs watercress to garnish

Heat the oil in a saucepan. Add the carrots and leeks, cover and
sweat over a low heat for 15 minutes. Add the potato slices, pepper
to taste and 300 ml (½ pint) of the stock. Bring to the boil and simmer
until the potatoes are soft. Liquidize and return to the saucepan,
adding the remaining stock and the milk. Adjust the seasoning and
serve hot or cold with watercress to garnish.

## Chicken, Spinach and Sweetcorn Soup
### SERVES 4

2 chicken breasts, skinned and each chopped into 8 pieces
600 ml (1 pint) water
2 tsp sunflower oil
1 onion, finely chopped
150 g (5 oz) spinach, stalks removed and leaves shredded
50 g (2 oz) canned sweetcorn
freshly ground black pepper
600 ml (1 pint) soya milk

Place the chicken and water in a saucepan, bring to the boil and simmer for 45 minutes. Heat the oil and gently fry the onions for 2 minutes until translucent. Remove the onions with a slotted spoon and add to the chicken liquid. Add the spinach and sweetcorn. Season with black pepper to taste, and cook for a further 5 minutes. Add the milk and heat through before serving.

## *Main courses*

## Chicken and Sweetcorn Risotto
### SERVES 4

1 tbsp vegetable oil
50 g (2 oz) finely chopped onion
225 g (8 oz) long grain brown rice
600 ml (1 pint) chicken stock
100 g (4 oz) frozen peas
100 g (4 oz) frozen sweetcorn
175 g (6 oz) cooked chicken, diced
pepper
dried mixed herbs

Heat the oil and cook the onion for 2-3 minutes without colouring. Add the rice and cook for another 2-3 minutes. Add the stock, bring to the boil and simmer for 15 minutes. Add the chicken, peas and sweetcorn. Bring back to the boil. Simmer until the rice is cooked and the stock is absorbed. Season with pepper and the mixed herbs, and serve.

## Broccoli and Sweetcorn Stuffed Plaice

SERVES 4

4 plaice fillets
freshly ground black pepper

*For the stuffing*
50 g (2 oz) broccoli tops
50 g (2 oz) cooked brown rice
25 g (1 oz) canned sweetcorn
1 tbsp fresh lemon juice
parsley to garnish

Preheat the oven to Gas Mark 4 (180°C, 350°F). Skin the plaice fillets and sprinkle them with black pepper. Cook the broccoli tops for 5 minutes, drain well and chop. Place the broccoli, rice and sweetcorn in a bowl and mix well with the lemon juice. Divide the mixture between the 4 plaice fillets, roll up and secure each with a cocktail stick.

Place in an ovenproof dish, cover and bake for 25-30 minutes, until the fish is tender. Remove the cocktail sticks and garnish with parsley before serving on a warm plate.

## Liver and Sweetcorn

SERVES 2

1 tbsp sunflower oil
50 g (2 oz) onions, chopped
1 small clove garlic, crushed
300 g (10 oz) liver
100 g (4 oz) canned sweetcorn
4 tbsp vegetable stock
pinch of thyme
freshly ground black pepper to taste

Heat the oil in a frying pan and add the onions and garlic. Fry gently for about 2 minutes, until the onions are soft. Add the liver and cook, turning occasionally, until browned. Add the sweetcorn and cook for 1 minute longer. Stir in the remaining ingredients and bring to the boil. Reduce the heat, cover and simmer for 2 minutes.

## Corn Pasta with Mince and Spinach
### SERVES 4

115 g (4 oz) soya mince (textured vegetable protein)
200 ml (7 fl oz) vegetable stock
4 servings Tomato Sauce (see below)
275 g (10 oz) corn pasta
150 g (5 oz) spinach, stalks removed and leaves shredded
4 sprigs coriander to garnish

Cook the soya mince in vegetable stock together with the tomato sauce. Simmer for 10 minutes. Cook the pasta in boiling water as directed on the packet. Add the spinach to the soya mince mixture and simmer for 2 minutes. Drain the pasta, divide into 4 dishes and pour over the sauce. Top with sprigs of coriander and serve.

## Root Veggie Bake
### SERVES 4

450 g (1 lb) potatoes, scrubbed and sliced
175 g (6 oz) carrots, scrubbed and sliced
175 g (6 oz) parsnips, scrubbed and sliced
1 tbsp almond pieces
1 tbsp fresh parsley, chopped
4 servings Tomato Sauce (see below)

Bring the potatoes, carrots and parsnips to the boil in a pan of water. Simmer for 10 minutes, then drain. Heat through the tomato sauce. In a large greased ovenproof dish, layer the potatoes, carrots, parsnips, almonds, parsley and tomato sauce. Bake in a preheated oven at Gas Mark 4 (180°C, 350°F) for 15 minutes. Serve immediately.

## Tomato Sauce
### MAKES 4 SERVINGS

2 tsp olive oil
100 g (4 oz) onion, finely chopped
1 clove garlic, crushed
400 g (14 oz) fresh ripe tomatoes, chopped and skins removed *or*
a 400 g (14 oz) can plum tomatoes, drained and chopped
2 tsp dried mixed herbs *or* fresh basil, chopped
freshly ground black pepper to taste

Heat the oil, add the onion and garlic, cover, and cook gently for 5 minutes until the onion is soft. Add the tomatoes and herbs. Cover and cook for 15 minutes. Season with freshly ground black pepper. Cool, if serving the sauce as a salad dressing.

This sauce can be kept in a refrigerator for 4 days.

## Potato and Rice Bread

MAKES 2 LOAVES

275 g (10 oz) potato flour
225g (8 oz) brown rice flour
1½ packets easy blend yeast
1 tsp sugar
1 tbsp oil
½-1 tsp salt
300-350 ml (10-12 fl oz) hand-hot water

Mix together flours and yeast. Add the sugar, oil and salt and mix to a thick batter with hand-hot water. Grease two 450g (1lb) loaf tins. Divide the mixture between the two tins, cover and leave to rise in a warm place for 20-30 minutes. Bake the loaves in a preheated oven at Gas Mark 8 (230°C, 450°F) for 35-40 minutes. The bread will slightly contract from the sides of the tin when cooked. Cool for 5 minutes in the tin and turn out on to a wire rack. Slice when cold.

# 19

# Phase 3
# citrus week

## _____ Fast options _____

### *Lunches*

Mackerel and salad
Pilchards and salad
Sardines and salad
Tuna and salad

Prawn and Rice Salad (page 117)
Rice salad with chicken
Rice salad with nuts

Avocado and salad

Chicken and salad
Ham and salad
Turkey and salad

Followed by fresh fruit salad with nuts and soya yoghurt *or* citrus
    fruit salad with nuts and yoghurt
Grapefruit segments
Orange and Cucumber Salad (page 151)

### *Dinner*

Chicken with vegetables and rice
Lamb chops and vegetables
Steak and vegetables
Grilled plaice with vegetables and rice
Steamed salmon with vegetables and rice
Stir-fried vegetables and rice with prawns, nuts or chicken
Tomato omelette with vegetables
Prawns and egg salad
Cold meat salad
Grilled fish with rice and salad

Fresh oranges
Fruit salad *or* Citrus Fruit Salad (page 152)
Fresh orange juice *or* fresh grapefruit juice
Orange and Lemon Sorbet (page 154)
Lemon tea

## *Drinks and snacks*

### Hot drinks

Chicory
2 cups of coffee (if no diarrhoea)
Dandelion coffee (boiled root) or instant dandelion coffee (if not
    intolerant to lactose)
Fruit teas
Orange and lemon herbal teas
Rooibosch, Eleven O'clock tea (especially good for gut spasm)
2 cups of tea (if not constipated)

### Cold drinks

Avoid alcohol
Apple juice/Appletise
Bottled water (with or without gas)
Citrus Spring
Grapefruit juice
Lemon juice
Orange juice (from a carton or freshly squeezed)
Tonic water

### Snacks

Baked Apple (page 125) or pear
Citrus Fruit Salad (page 152)
Coconut Rounds (page 125)
Fruit sorbet (see recipes, pages 126, 153 and 154)
Fruity Ginger Salad (page 153)
Gooseberry Jelly
Non-citrus fruits
Oranges
Rice cakes, with sugar-free jam or mashed banana or hazelnut or
    almond butter
Rice salad
Soya ice cream
Soya yoghurt
Tangerines

# Menus

## *Day 1*

### Breakfast

½ grapefruit
Rice Krispies with chopped fruit and nuts and soya milk
Rice cakes *or* rice bread (toasted) with butter and sugar-free jam

### Lunch

Canned sardines
Watercress, Fennel and Lemon Salad (page 151)
Jacket potato

### Dinner

Lemon steaks
Chips
French beans
Green salad

Citrus Fruit Salad (page 152)

## *Day 2*

### Breakfast

Grapefruit and Orange Salad (page 151)
Rice bread (toasted) with butter and sugar-free jam

### Lunch

Chicken drumstick
Orange and Cucumber Salad (page 151)
Jacket potato

### Dinner

Mackerel with Lemon Stuffing (page 149)
Spinach
Carrots

Fruity Ginger Salad (page 153)

## *Day 3*

### Breakfast
2 poached eggs and tomatoes with rice bread (toasted) and butter

### Lunch
Lean ham
Green salad
Rice salad

Fresh orange

### Dinner
Chicken and rice salad
Jacket potato

Pineapple in Orange Juice (page 152)

## *Day 4*

### Breakfast
½ grapefruit
Cornflakes and soya milk
Rice bread (toasted) with butter and sugar-free jam

### Lunch
Mackerel in tomato sauce
Watercress, Fennel and Lemon Salad (page 151)

Fresh orange

### Dinner
Halibut Fruit (page 150)
Rice
Courgettes
Mange-touts

## *Day 5*

### Breakfast
Grapefruit and Orange Salad (page 151) with chopped nuts and
soya yoghurt
Rice bread (toasted) with sugar-free jam

## Lunch

Fish Balls (page 118)
Green salad
Coleslaw

## Dinner

Liver with Orange (page 149)
Mashed potatoes
Spring greens
Baked onions

Orange Snow (page 152)

## *Day 6*

## Breakfast

2 scrambled eggs and tomatoes on rice bread (toasted)

## Lunch

Grilled mackerel with Orange and Herb Sauce (page 150)
Green salad

## Dinner

Tarragon and Orange Chicken (page 147)
Cauliflower
Sweetcorn
Roast potatoes

Colada Sorbet (page 153)

## *Day 7*

## Breakfast

Grapefruit and Orange Salad (page 151), soya yoghurt, chopped
  nuts
Rice bread (toasted) with butter and sugar-free jam

## Lunch

Canned tuna in brine
Orange and Cucumber Salad (page 151)
Jacket potato

## Dinner

Ham Steaks with Orange Sauce (page 148)
Cabbage
Mashed potatoes
Peas

Orange and Lemon Sorbet (page 154)

―――――――――― Recipes ――――――――――

### *Main courses*

### Tarragon and Orange Chicken

SERVES 4

1 tbsp vegetable oil
4 chicken breasts, boned and skinned
8 shallots, finely chopped
2 oranges
150 ml (¼ pint) chicken stock
½ tsp tomato purée
1 tbsp chopped fresh tarragon
freshly ground black pepper to taste

Heat the oil in a frying pan and brown the chicken and shallots on all sides. Finely grate the rind of one orange, then peel both oranges and remove the white pith. Remove all membranes from the fruit segments and reserve any fruit juices. Mix together the rind, juice, stock and purée and add to the pan. Cover and simmer gently for 15 minutes turning the chicken breasts twice. Add the orange segments, tarragon and seasoning. Warm through gently.

Slice and fan out the chicken breasts, then spoon the oranges and shallots over the chicken. Cook the sauce until it is reduced to a syrup. Spoon over the chicken and serve with boiled rice.

# Lemon Steaks

SERVES 4

4 sirloin steaks
grated rind and juice of ½ lemon
3 tbsp chopped fresh parsley
2 tbsp beef stock
1 tsp tomato purée
2 tbsp olive oil
2 tbsp polyunsaturated margarine
1 tsp French mustard
1 clove garlic, crushed
freshly ground black pepper

Trim any excess fat from the steaks. Mix together the rind, lemon juice, parsley, stock and tomato purée, and set aside.

In a large frying pan, combine the oil, margarine, mustard, garlic and pepper. Stir well and heat until the mixture begins to bubble.

Gently fry the steaks in the seasoned mixture for 3-4 minutes, turning them half way. Pour over the reserved mixture and cook for a further 2-3 minutes or until cooked to taste (you may wish to adjust the cooking times according to personal preference for rare, medium or well-done steaks). Serve with a mixed salad and sauté potatoes.

# Ham Steaks with Orange Sauce

SERVES 2

100 ml (4 fl oz) orange juice
1 orange, peeled and chopped
1 tsp cornflour
4 tbsp water
lemon juice to taste
2 × 100 g (4 oz) ham steaks
sprigs of parsley and twists of orange to garnish

Pour the orange juice into a pan and add the chopped orange.

Blend the cornflour to a paste with water. Stir into the orange juice and flesh mixture. Bring to the boil, stirring continuously. Reduce the heat and simmer for 2 minutes. Add the lemon juice.

While the sauce is simmering, grill the ham steaks for 7-8 minutes, turning once. Pour the orange sauce over the ham steaks. Serve garnished with sprigs of parsley and twists of orange.

## Liver with Orange

SERVES 2

1 tbsp oil
1 small onion, thinly sliced
170 g (6 oz) lambs' liver, thinly sliced
1 tbsp flour, seasoned with freshly ground black pepper
½ green pepper, cored and diced
1 × 75 g (3 oz) rasher of lean bacon, sliced into 2.5 cm (1 inch) pieces
100 ml (4 fl oz) orange juice
2 oranges, separated into segments and halved

Heat the oil and gently fry the onion for 2-5 minutes. Toss the liver in the seasoned flour and place the liver, bacon and pepper in the pan with the onion and fry for a further minute. Stir in the orange juice and simmer for 5 minutes. Add the halved orange segments, heat through for 1 minute and serve.

## Mackerel with Lemon Stuffing

SERVES 4

4 × 175 g (6 oz) mackerel, split and boned
juice of half a lemon
freshly ground black pepper
3 tbsp water
4 slices lemon to garnish

*Stuffing*
2 tsp sunflower oil
1 small onion, finely chopped
125 g (4 oz) cooked brown rice
finely grated rind and juice of 1 lemon
1 tbsp fresh chopped parsley
1 small egg, beaten

Preheat the oven to Gas Mark 3 (160°C, 325°F).

To prepare the stuffing, heat the oil in a pan, add the onion and cook for 5 minutes or until golden. Transfer to a mixing bowl and combine with the remaining stuffing ingredients.

Place the mackerel on a flat surface and sprinkle the flesh with lemon juice and black pepper. Spoon the stuffing into the fish and re-shape. Place in an ovenproof dish and add the 3 tbsp of water. Cover and bake for 15-20 minutes. Garnish with the lemon slices, before serving.

## Halibut Fruit

SERVES 2

grated rind and juice of 2 oranges and 1 lemon
1 orange, peeled and separated into segments
2 halibut steaks, cut in half
extra orange and lemon slices to garnish

Place the grated rinds in an ovenproof dish with the juices. Add the fish and baste well. This can be left to marinate for 1-6 hours, turning occasionally. Cover the dish with foil and bake in a preheated oven at Gas Mark 4 (180°C, 350°F) for 10 minutes. Add the orange segments and bake for a further 10 minutes. Serve garnished with the orange and lemon slices.

## Orange and Herb Sauce

SERVES 4

2 tsp sunflower oil
1 small onion, finely chopped
175 ml (6 fl oz) frozen concentrated orange juice
2 tsp chopped tarragon
2 tsp chopped parsley
freshly ground black pepper to taste
2 tsp cornflour
1 tbsp water
1 orange, peeled, separated into segments, pith removed and chopped

Heat the oil and gently fry the onions. Add the orange juice, herbs and black pepper. Bring to the boil and simmer for 2-3 minutes.

Mix the cornflour with the water and stir into the sauce, bringing slowly to the boil and stirring constantly. Add the chopped orange segments, heat for 1-2 minutes and serve.

This sauce can be used to complement meat, fish or vegetable dishes. It can be made in larger quantities in advance and frozen.

## Orange and Cucumber Salad

SERVES 4

2 oranges, peeled and separated into segments
½ cucumber, thinly sliced
1 small onion, thinly sliced into rings
½ small lettuce

Mix all the ingredients together.

## Grapefruit and Orange Salad

SERVES 4

1 whole grapefruit
1 orange
75 g (3 oz) sunflower seeds
50 g (2 oz) mixed nuts, chopped
orange juice, freshly squeezed

Remove the rind of the grapefruit and orange and chop the flesh.
Mix with the sunflower seeds and nuts and a little orange juice.

## Watercress, Fennel and Lemon Salad

SERVES 4

1 large fennel bulb, thinly sliced
1 small bunch watercress, washed and trimmed
1 handful fresh parsley, washed, well dried and finely chopped
freshly ground black pepper to taste
1 tbsp fresh lemon juice
1 lemon

Mix together the fennel, watercress and parsley. Add the black
pepper and lemon juice. Thinly slice the lemon, cut each slice into
segments and add to the salad.

# *Desserts*

## Orange Snow

SERVES 4

300 ml (½ pint) cold water
15 g (½ oz) powdered gelatine
50 g (2 oz) caster sugar
thinly pared rind and juice of 1 orange
3 egg whites

Pour the water into a saucepan and sprinkle the gelatine on top.
Leave to soak for 5 minutes. Stir in the sugar and orange rind. Place
the pan over low heat and stir until both the gelatine and sugar have
dissolved. DO NOT ALLOW TO BOIL. Strain the mixture into a
large bowl and set aside until cold. Stand the bowl in a basin of cold
water and ice cubes. Strain the orange juice and add to the gelatine
mixture along with the egg whites. Using a rotary beater beat the
mixture until it is thick and white. Chill before serving.

## Citrus Fruit Salad

SERVES 4

4 medium oranges
2 large pink grapefruit
4 tbsp clear honey
2 bananas

Peel the oranges and grapefruit, removing the rind, pith and fine
skin. Separate the segments using a sharp knife. Put the fruit in a
bowl, adding any juice extracted by squeezing the skins. Fold in the
honey and chill for 10 minutes. Peel and slice the bananas and fold
into the fruit just before serving.

## Pineapple in Orange Sauce

SERVES 4

1 medium pineapple
25 g (1 oz) polyunsaturated margarine
90 ml (3 fl oz) unsweetened orange juice
40 g (1½ oz) Barbados sugar

Remove the foliage and husk from the pineapple. Slice the flesh into 8 rings and remove the cores. Preheat the grill on Moderate and place the pineapple on to a heatproof dish. Melt the margarine in a saucepan over a low heat. Remove before it foams and brush the pineapple rings with it. Put the orange juice and sugar into a saucepan and stir over a low heat until the sugar dissolves. Spoon the liquid over the pineapple. Place the dish under the grill about 5 cm (2 inches) from the heat and cook for 2 minutes on each side. Serve immediately.

## Fruity Ginger Salad

### SERVES 4

2 apricots
2 eating apples
1 orange
250ml (8 fl oz) low-calorie ginger ale
50 g (2 oz) seedless grapes
2 bananas
2 tbsp lemon juice

Plunge the apricots into a bowl of boiling water for 30 seconds. Drain and peel. Halve the apricots, remove the stones and dice the flesh. Core and dice the apples, leaving on the skin. Peel the orange and divide into segments. Discard all the white pith. Put the apricot, apple and orange into a serving bowl with the ginger ale. Stir lightly, cover and leave for 1 hour. Meanwhile, cut the grapes in half. Peel and slice the bananas and mix them with the lemon juice to prevent discolouration. Add the bananas and grapes to the other fruit. Serve in individual glasses or bowls.

## Colada Sorbet

### SERVES 4

450 ml (¾ pint) pineapple juice
300 ml (½ pint) water
100 g (4 oz) caster sugar
4 tsp grated lemon rind
3 tbsp lemon juice
50 g (2 oz) creamed coconut
2 egg whites

Pour the pineapple juice and water into a saucepan and add the sugar, rind and lemon juice. Heat gently until the sugar has dissolved. Increase the heat and cook rapidly until it threads. (Remove a little syrup with a spoon and allow it to fall on to a dish. The syrup should form a fine thread. If you have a sugar thermometer, the heat should be 107°C or 225°F.) Remove from the heat and immediately add the creamed coconut, stirring gently until it melts. Allow to cool. Pour into a rigid freezeproof container and freeze for 1½ hours. Stir occasionally until mushy. Whisk the egg whites until they form soft peaks. Fold into the mix and freeze for a further 3 hours, beating the mixture twice at hourly intervals.

## Orange and Lemon Sorbet

SERVES 4

2 large oranges
1 lemon
450 ml (¾ pint) water
concentrated apple juice to taste
3 tbsp natural yoghurt
2 egg whites
peeled orange segments to garnish

Thinly pare the rind from the oranges and lemon and place the rind together with the water in a saucepan. Simmer gently for 8 minutes, and strain into a bowl.

Cut the fruit in half and squeeze out the juice.

Add the orange and lemon juice to the liquid from the orange and lemon rind and place into a bowl. Stir in the apple juice to taste. Pour the orange and lemon liquid into a shallow freezer container and freeze until semi-frozen.

Turn the semi-frozen orange and lemon mixture into a bowl and beat to break up the crystals. Mix in the yoghurt.

Whisk the egg white until stiff and gently fold into the orange and lemon and yoghurt mixture. Return to the freezer until firm. Scoop the sorbet into dessert glasses and garnish with peeled orange segments before serving.

# 20
# Phase 4
# dairy week

## Joanna's story

Joanna Jones had suffered with IBS for as long as she could remember.

'According to my mother my symptoms started shortly after I was weaned. I suffered with agonizing stomach cramps which as I got older got gradually worse. I used to end up curled up in a ball on my mum's knee writhing in pain, two or three times a week. I went to numerous doctors, and was continually having tests and investigations, all of which proved negative. They concluded that it was all in my mind, and that time would heal all wounds.

'By the time I was ten my mother rebelled against their diagnosis of "all in the mind", and insisted I was investigated in hospital. After a brief examination, it was decided that I had a "dry bowel" and that I should eat a high-fibre diet, with loads of porridge and wholemeal bread. The pains continued to get worse, and I remember one trip home from school, when I was unable to walk for pain, so I sat on the pavement for an hour until it had subsided.

'My mum suggested that the pains might be food related, and suspected milk, as I had had the pains when she introduced milk to my diet when I was a baby. She took me off all dairy products and the pains disappeared totally. We gradually introduced dairy products, until we got to milk, and then the pains returned.

'I now manage to drink skimmed milk in small quantities, and avoid other dairy products where possible. The pains only return if I drink lots of skimmed milk, or even a small amount of full-fat milk.'

# Fast options

## *Lunches*

Mackerel and salad
Pilchards and salad
Sardines and salad
Tuna and salad

Prawn and Rice Salad (page 117)
Rice salad with chicken
Rice salad with nuts

Avocado and salad

Chicken and salad
Ham and salad
Turkey and salad

Banana milk shake (home-made)
Cheese and rice cakes
Cheese omelette
Cheese on rice bread, toasted
Cheese salad
Fruit salad with fruit yoghurt
Greek Salad (page 168)
Jacket potato with grated cheese

## *Dinner*

Chicken with vegetables and rice
Lamb chops and vegetables
Steak and vegetables
Grilled plaice with vegetables and rice
Steamed salmon with vegetables and rice
Stir-fried vegetables and rice, with prawns, nuts or chicken
Tomato omelette with vegetables
Prawn and egg salad
Cold meat salad
Grilled fish, rice and salad
Cauliflower cheese (using rice flour)
Spaghetti Bolognese (with rice or corn spaghetti or noodles) with
    grated cheese or Parmesan cheese

Corn pasta, canned tomatoes, basil and Parmesan cheese
Grilled sliced courgettes, fresh tomatoes and Cheddar cheese
Omelette, jacket potato or Greek Salad (page 168) [as listed for
    lunch]

Baked egg custard
Fruit salad and cream
Rice pudding
Strawberries and cream
Yoghurt and fruit

## *Drinks and snacks*

(Use cow's milk.)

### Hot drinks

Chicory
2 cups of coffee (if no diarrhoea)
Dandelion coffee (boiled root) or instant dandelion coffee (if not
    intolerant to lactose)
Herbal teas, including fruit teas
Rooibosch, Eleven O'clock tea (especially good for gut spasm)
2 cups of tea (if not constipated)

### Cold drinks

Avoid alcohol
Apple juice/Appletise
Bottled water (with or without gas)
Milk
Milk shake
Tonic water

### Snacks

Baked Apple (page 125) or pear
Cheese and apple
Coconut Rounds (page 125)
Dips – hummus or taramasalata
Fruit fool (non-citrus)
Fruit mousse (non-citrus)
Fruit salad (without citrus fruit)
Fruit sorbet (see recipes, pages 126, 153 and 154)
Gooseberry Jelly
Greek Salad (page 168)

Ice cream
Non-citrus fruits
Rice cakes, with sugar-free jam or mashed banana or hazelnut or almond butter
Rice pudding
Rice salad
Soya ice cream
Soya yoghurt
Yoghurt

# Menus

## *Day 1*

### Breakfast

Cornflakes
Fruit, nuts and cow's milk
Rice cakes *or* rice bread (toasted) with sugar-free jam and butter

### Lunch

Grated cheese
Courgette and Cauliflower Salad (page 124)
Jacket potato

### Dinner

Spinach and Egg Bake (page 166)
Jacket potato
Carrots

Blackberries and Hazelnut Cheese (page 170)

## *Day 2*

### Breakfast

Fruit salad with chopped nuts and yoghurt
Rice cakes *or* rice bread (toasted) with butter and sugar-free jam

### Lunch

Ricotta Stuffed Courgettes (page 167)
Green salad

### Dinner

Plaice with Yoghurt and Nuts (page 164)
Spinach and rice

Passion Fruit Fool (page 169)

## *Day 3*

### Breakfast

2 poached eggs and grilled tomatoes with rice bread (toasted)

### Lunch

Turkey breast
Mixed salad
Jacket potato and soured cream

### Dinner

Speedy Vegetable Soufflé (page 165)
Mange-touts
Carrots
Cauliflower

Apple custard

## *Day 4*

### Breakfast

Rice Krispies with chopped fruit and nuts and cow's milk
Rice bread (toasted) with butter and sugar-free jam

### Lunch

Carrot and Courgette Soup (page 162)
Root vegetable salad

### Dinner

Trout with Mustard Sauce (page 164)
Mashed potatoes
Peas
Green beans

Rice pudding

## *Day 5*

### Breakfast

2 egg cheese omelette
Rice bread (toasted) with butter and sugar-free jam

### Lunch

Greek Salad (page 168)
Nachips (corn chips)

### Dinner

Cheesy Brown Rice Pie (page 163)
Courgettes
Carrots

Strawberry Cheesecake (page 168)

## *Day 6*

### Breakfast

Chopped fruit and nuts and natural yoghurt
Rice bread (toasted) with butter and sugar-free jam

### Lunch

Lentil Soup (page 161)
Jacket potato and grated cheese

### Dinner

Yoghurt Roast Chicken (page 163)
Rice
Mange-touts
Cauliflower

Gooseberry mousse

## *Day 7*

### Breakfast

½ grapefruit
2 rounds of cheese on rice bread (toasted)

## Lunch
Potato and Cheese Bake (page 165)
Green salad

## Dinner
Beef Stroganoff (page 162)
Mashed potatoes
Carrots

Strawberry Cream (page 168) and fresh fruit

_____ **Recipes** _____

### *Soups*

### Lentil Soup
SERVES 4

50 g (2 oz) butter
1 carrot, chopped
1 onion, chopped
¼ turnip, diced
1 large potato, diced
100 g (4 oz) lentils
2 tbsp chopped fresh parsley
600 ml (1 pint) milk
300 ml (½ pint) chicken stock
freshly ground black pepper
150 ml (¼ pint) single cream

Melt the butter in a pan and gently fry the vegetables for 10 minutes.
Add the lentils, parsley, milk and stock, and season with pepper.
Bring to the boil, cover and simmer for 1 hour. Cool slightly, liquidize
and stir in the cream. Serve hot.

## Carrot and Courgette Soup

SERVES 4

50 g (2 oz) butter
1 onion, chopped
225 g (8 oz) carrots, chopped
225 g (8 oz) courgettes, chopped
40 g (1½ oz) cornflour
450 ml (¾ pint) chicken stock
450 ml (¾ pint) milk (or soya milk)
freshly ground black pepper
pinch of nutmeg
75 g (3 oz) Cheddar cheese, grated

Melt the butter in a pan, then add the onion, carrots and courgettes.
Cover and cook for 5 minutes over a low heat until soft. Add the
flour, then gradually blend in the stock and milk. Season and add nutmeg, bring to the boil and simmer for 20 minutes. Liquidize the soup
and serve hot sprinkled with grated cheese.

## *Main courses*

### Beef Stroganoff

SERVES 4

2 tsp oil
25 g (1 oz) butter
1 medium onion, finely sliced
100 g (4 oz) red pepper chopped
½ beef stock cube
150 ml (¼ pint) boiling water
1 level tsp tomato purée
450 g (1 lb) fillet of beef, cut into thin strips
6 level tbsp soured cream
freshly ground black pepper to taste

Heat half the oil and half the butter in a non-stick frying pan. Add the
onion, and cook over a low heat, stirring frequently until soft. Stir in
the peppers.

Dissolve the stock cube in the water, stir in the tomato purée,
then add to the pan. Boil rapidly until the liquid is reduced to about 50
ml (2 fl oz). Tip the reduced liquid into a bowl and set aside.

Heat the remaining oil and butter in the pan and add the meat, which should all fit easily in the pan in a single layer. If necessary, cook in 2 batches. Cook over a fairly high heat for about 3 minutes on each side until the outsides are browned. Shake and toss the pan frequently as the meat cooks. Add the vegetable mixture and heat through. Stir in the soured cream and season. Heat through but do not boil. Serve immediately.

## Cheesy Brown Rice Pie

### SERVES 6

170 g (5½ oz) brown rice, cooked
250 g (8 oz) mature Cheddar, grated
4 tbsp Parmesan cheese
2 spring onions, chopped
2 courgettes, grated
1 red pepper, diced
315 g (10 oz) tin cut asparagus, drained and chopped
3 tbsp pine nuts, toasted
3 eggs, lightly beaten
200 g (6½ oz) natural yoghurt
Salt and black pepper

Preheat the oven to Gas Mark 5 (190°C, 375°F).

Combine all the ingredients in a bowl and mix well. Season to taste. Turn the mixture into a greased 23 cm (9 inch) spring-form tin.

Bake for 40 minutes until firm and golden. Leave in the tin for 5 minutes before removing.

Serve hot or cold. Ideal for picnics.

## Yoghurt Roast Chicken

### SERVES 4

225 ml (8 fl oz) natural yoghurt
2 tsp curry powder (mild, medium or hot as preferred)
½ bunch fresh coriander, finely chopped
1 tbsp grated fresh root ginger
3 garlic cloves, crushed
1 × 1.5-1.75 kg (3-4 lb) oven-ready chicken

Combine the yoghurt, curry powder, coriander, ginger and garlic. Rub all over the chicken, cover and set aside for 1-2 hours.

Place the chicken in a roasting tin with the yoghurt sauce and bake in a preheated oven at Gas Mark 4 (180°C, 350°F) for 1¼-1½ hours.

Transfer the chicken to a serving dish and keep warm. Stir together the remaining chicken juices and yoghurt sauce in the roasting tin and boil rapidly to reduce, if necessary. Serve the chicken with the sauce.

## Trout with Mustard Sauce

### SERVES 4

4 rainbow trout (350 g/12 oz each), cleaned
freshly ground black pepper
2 tbsp vegetable oil
50 g (2 oz) butter
4 tbsp chopped onion
150 ml (¼ pint) single cream
about 3 tsp Dijon mustard
1 tsp lemon juice
1 lemon and parsley to garnish

Heat the grill to Moderate. Pat the trout dry and season them inside. Then brush them with half of the oil and grill for 5 minutes each side until cooked right through.

Meanwhile, heat the butter with the remaining oil in a frying pan, add the onion and cook until softened. Stir in the cream, mustard to taste, lemon juice and seasoning. Cook gently for 2-3 minutes without boiling. Place the trout on a warm serving dish. Spoon over the sauce and serve with lemon wedges and parsley.

## Plaice with Yoghurt and Nuts

### SERVES 4

750 g (1½ lb) plaice fillets
2 bananas, sliced
75 g (3 oz) almonds
25 g (1 oz) chopped almonds to garnish

*sauce*
50 g (2 oz) margarine
50 g (2 oz) cornflour
300 ml (½ pint) milk
3 tbsp natural yoghurt
freshly ground black pepper to taste

Place the fish in a greased, shallow ovenproof dish. Cover and bake in preheated oven at Gas Mark 4 (180°C, 350°F) for 10 minutes. Remove the fish from the oven and arrange the banana and almonds over the fish.

Melt the margarine in a pan and stir in the cornflour. Cook for 1 minute and gradually add the milk until the sauce thickens. Remove from the heat and stir in the yoghurt.

Season the fish with the black pepper.

Pour the sauce over the fish and return to the oven for 15 minutes. Garnish with the chopped almonds.

## Speedy Vegetable Soufflé

SERVES 4

225 g (8 oz) cooked potatoes
50 g (2 oz) cooked cauliflower
50 g (2 oz) cooked Brussels sprouts
50 g (2 oz) cooked swede
50 g (2 oz) cooked carrots
1 tbsp cream
3 eggs, separated
100 g (4 oz) hard cheese, grated
freshly ground black pepper

Preheat the oven to Gas Mark 7 (220°C, 425°F). Lightly grease an 18 cm (7 inch) soufflé dish with butter or margarine. In a bowl finely mash together all the vegetables and beat in the cream, egg yolks and cheese. Season to taste.

Whisk the egg whites stiffly. Lightly but thoroughly fold them into the vegetable and cream mixture. Spoon into the prepared dish and bake for 20 minutes or until well risen and lightly coloured on top. Serve immediately with salad.

## Potato and Cheese Bake

SERVES 4

750 g (1½ lb) potatoes, peeled
50 g (2 oz) polyunsaturated margarine
2 medium onions, finely chopped
25 g (1 oz) cornflour
freshly ground black pepper to taste
½ tsp dried mixed herbs
350 ml (12 fl oz) milk
225 g (8 oz) Cheddar cheese, finely grated

Preheat the oven to Gas Mark 4 (180°C, 350°F).

Boil and mash the potatoes. Place them in a medium mixing bowl and set aside.

Lightly grease a medium ovenproof dish with a teaspoon of the margarine.

Melt the remaining margarine in a saucepan over a moderate heat. Add the onions and fry until soft and golden. Remove the pan from the heat and using a wooden spoon stir in the cornflour, black pepper and herbs to make a smooth paste. Gradually add the milk, stirring constantly and taking care to avoid lumps. Return the pan to a low heat, stirring constantly, for 4-5 minutes or until the sauce is smooth and thick. Add 175 g (6 oz) of the cheese and cook until it has melted, stirring all the time. Gradually pour the cheese sauce over the potatoes, beating constantly with a wooden spoon until the mixture is smooth.

Turn the mixture into the prepared dish and smooth down with the back of a spoon. Sprinkle with the remaining cheese. Place the dish in the centre of the oven and bake for 20-25 minutes or until the top is golden brown. Serve immediately.

### Spinach and Egg Bake

SERVES 2

350 g (12 oz) frozen chopped spinach
2 eggs
8 tsp single cream
freshly ground black pepper to taste
25 g (1 oz) low-fat cottage cheese, grated

Preheat the oven to Gas Mark 4 (180°C, 350°F).

Boil the spinach, according to the instructions on the packet. Press into a sieve to drain the excess water. Divide the spinach between two dishes and make a deep well in the centre. Break an egg into each well.

Spoon 4 teaspoons of cream over each egg and season well with pepper. Bake for 20 minutes. Remove from the oven, sprinkle with the cheese and place under a grill for 1-2 minutes. Serve immediately.

## Ricotta Stuffed Courgettes

SERVES 4

8 medium courgettes
freshly ground black pepper
2 tbsp olive oil
1 medium onion, finely chopped
1 clove garlic, crushed
175 g (6 oz) ricotta cheese
2 tsp dried basil
1 (400 g/14 oz) can chopped tomatoes
1 medium onion, finely chopped
1 tsp dried mixed herbs
3 tbsp wheat-free breadcrumbs
fresh basil sprigs to garnish

Score the courgettes lengthways with the prongs of a fork and then cut in half lengthways. Scoop out the flesh and reserve leaving a thin margin of flesh so that the skin does not break. Blanch the courgette shells in boiling water for 10 minutes. Drain, then stand skin-side up on absorbent paper.

Heat the oil in a frying pan, add the medium chopped onion, garlic and reserved courgette flesh. Fry gently for 5 minutes until soft and lightly coloured. Turn into a bowl and add the ricotta and basil. Season with black pepper and stir well. Fill the courgette shells equally with the ricotta mixture. Gently fry the remaining onion in a frying pan until soft, add the tomatoes and fry for 1 minute. Pour into the bottom of an ovenproof dish which is large enough to hold the courgettes in a single layer. Place the courgettes side by side on top of the sauce, with the filling face upwards, and sprinkle with wheat-free breadcrumbs. Bake in the oven at Gas Mark 6 (200°C, 400°F) for 20 minutes. Serve hot, garnished with plenty of basil sprigs.

## Greek Salad

SERVES 4

½ cucumber, thickly sliced
1 small onion, sliced
4 large tomatoes, sliced
4 black olives
100 g (4 oz) feta cheese, drained and cut into squares
4 tbsp olive oil
1 tbsp lemon juice
2 tsp chopped fresh oregano
½ small iceberg lettuce, shredded

Cut the cucumber slices into quarters and place in a bowl with the onion, tomatoes, olives and cheese. Mix well. Combine the oil, lemon juice and oregano and blend together thoroughly. Place the lettuce in a glass bowl and spoon the salad ingredients on top. Pour the dressing over.

## *Desserts*

## Strawberry Cheesecake

SERVES 6

*For the base*
100 g (4 oz) wheat-free digestive biscuits, crushed
25 g (1 oz) melted butter

*For the filling*
175 g (6 oz) strawberries, plus a few to decorate
50 g (2 oz) caster sugar
150 ml (¼ pint) double cream
100 g (4 oz) smooth cottage cheese
1 kiwi fruit, peeled and sliced

Mix the ingredients for the base together, press into a loose-bottomed cake tin and chill. Wash and hull the strawberries and mix with the caster sugar. Lightly whip the cream, then mix with the cottage cheese. Combine the strawberries and cream mixture and place on top of the base. Smooth out the surface and chill. Decorate with kiwi fruit and strawberries.

## Strawberry Cream

SERVES 6

100 g (4 oz) cottage cheese
150 ml (¼ pint) low-fat natural yoghurt
clear honey to taste
750 g (1½ lb) fresh strawberries, hulled

Purée the cottage cheese in a blender or food processor until smooth. Alternatively, push it through a fine wire sieve with the back of a spoon. In a bowl, beat the cheese and yoghurt together, with honey to taste. Set aside. Thinly slice the strawberries, reserving 6 for decoration. Distribute the sliced strawberries equally between 6 serving glasses. Pour the cheese mixture over the strawberries and chill in the fridge for 1 hour. Serve chilled with a whole strawberry on top for decoration.

## Passion Fruit Fool

SERVES 4

6 ripe passion fruit
150 ml (¼ pint) skimmed milk
2 tsp cornflour
2 tbsp water
150 ml (¼ pint) natural yoghurt
1 tbsp clear honey

Halve the passion fruit and scoop the fruit pulp into a bowl.
Gently heat the skimmed milk.
Blend cornflour and water into a smooth paste and then stir into hot milk. Stir over the heat until the sauce has thickened, remove to cool. Stir the yoghurt and honey into the sauce and leave until cool.
Combine the sauce and passion fruit pulp and spoon the mixture into serving dishes. Chill in the refrigerator for 3-4 hours before serving.

## Blackberries and Hazelnut Cheese

SERVES 6

750 g (1½ lb) fresh or frozen blackberries
1 tbsp dark brown sugar
½ tbsp tropical fruit juice
50 g (2 oz) hazelnuts
1 tsp caster sugar
175 g (6 oz) cottage cheese

Clean and prepare the blackberries. Mix together with the brown sugar and tropical fruit juice.

Toast the hazelnuts in a frying pan. When the nuts are brown, add the caster sugar. Shake the pan continuously to coat the nuts in the melting sugar. Set aside on a plate to cool.

Grind the caramel coated nuts and spread them out on a large sheet of greaseproof paper.

Roll the cottage cheese into 6 balls, then roll these into the crushed nuts gently pressing the nuts on to the surface of the cheese. Place the cheese balls on a plate and then into a refrigerator to set. To serve, place the individual cheese balls in dessert glasses and surround each one with the blackberries.

# 21

# Phase 5
# yeast week

## ───────── Fast options ─────────

### *Lunch*

Pilchards and salad
Mackerel and salad
Sardines and salad
Tuna and salad

Prawn and Rice Salad (page 117)
Rice salad with chicken
Rice salad with nuts

Avocado and salad

Chicken and salad
Ham and salad
Turkey and salad

Mushroom Omelette (page 182)
Blue-cheese salad
Yoghurt with nuts, seeds, fresh fruit and dried fruit
Dried Fruit Compôte (page 186)
Fruit with unsalted nuts and raisins (not peanuts)

### *Dinner*

Chicken with vegetables and rice
Lamb chops and vegetables
Steak and vegetables
Grilled plaice with vegetables and rice
Steamed salmon with vegetables and rice
Stir-fried vegetables and rice, with prawns, nuts or chicken
Tomato omelette with vegetables
Prawn and egg salad

Cold meat salad
Grilled fish, rice and salad
Stir-fried chicken, almonds and vegetables with soy sauce, red or
    white wine or brandy
Blue Chicken Salad (page 177)
Mushroom Omelette (page 182) with chips and salad

Dates, figs and other dried fruit
Fruit flambé (lightly poached fruit with orange juice, cream and
    liqueur)

## Drinks and snacks

### Hot drinks

Bovril or Marmite
Chicory
2 cups of coffee (if no diarrhoea)
Dandelion coffee (boiled root) or instant dandelion coffee (if not
    intolerant to lactose)
Herbal teas, including fruit teas
Rooibosch, Eleven O'clock tea (especially good for gut spasm)
2 cups of tea (if not constipated)

### Cold drinks

Apple juice/Appletise
Bottled water (with or without gas)
Tonic water

### Snacks

Apricot Cake (page 183)
Baked Apple (page 125) or pear
Coconut Rounds (page 125)
Dried apricots, figs, dates, mangoes or prunes
Dried Fruit Compôte (page 186) and soya ice cream
Fruit salad (without citrus fruit)
Fruit sorbet (see recipes, pages 126, 153 and 154)
Gooseberry Jelly
Non-citrus fruits
Pickled foods, gherkins, onions, herrings etc.
Raisins with almonds (if nuts don't upset you)
Rice cakes, with sugar-free jam or mashed banana or hazelnut or

almond butter
Rice salad
Soya ice cream
Soya yoghurt

## Menus

You are allowed 1-2 units of alcohol a day this week.
You may also put mayonnaise on your salads in yeast week.

### *Day 1*

**Breakfast**

Dried Fruit Compôte (page 186)
Rice bread (toasted) with butter and sugar-free jam

**Lunch**

Blue Chicken Salad (page 177)
Jacket potato

**Dinner**

Mushroom Omelette (page 182)
Chips
Peas

Apricot Cake (page 183)

### *Day 2*

**Breakfast**

Cornflakes, chopped nuts and raisins
Rice bread (toasted) with butter and sugar-free jam

**Lunch**

Chinese Tuna Salad (page 180)

**Dinner**

Chicken Pilaff (page 181)
Cauliflower
Carrots

Fruity Ginger Salad (page 153)

# *Day 3*

## Breakfast

Natural yoghurt with nuts and raisins and grated apple
Rice bread (toasted) with butter and sugar-free jam

## Lunch

Root Vegetable Soup (page 176)
Apple and Nut Salad (page 123)

## Dinner

Chicken Korma (page 176)
Rice
Spinach

Pear Paradise (page 185)

# *Day 4*

## Breakfast

Rice Krispies, figs and milk
Rice bread (toasted) with butter and sugar-free jam

## Lunch

Special Fried Rice (page 179)

## Dinner

Steak Kebabs and Barbecue Sauce (page 180)
Mixed Salad
Jacket potato

Brandied Apricot Flambé (page 185)

# *Day 5*

## Breakfast

Mushroom Omelette (page 182)
Rice bread (toasted) with butter and sugar-free jam

## Lunch

Japanese Sardines (page 178)
Green salad
Vinaigrette dressing

**Dinner**

Stuffed Marrow (page 182)
Mushrooms
Mixed salad

Carrot Cake (page 186)

## *Day 6*

**Breakfast**

Natural yoghurt with nuts, raisins and grated apples
Rice bread (toasted) with butter and sugar-free jam

**Lunch**

Seafood Salad (page 117) with vinaigrette dressing

**Dinner**

Lamb and Apricot Pilaff (page 115)
Cabbage
Cauliflower

Pears with Port and Orange Sauce (page 184)

## *Day 7*

**Breakfast**

Dried Fruit Compôte (page 186)
Cornflakes and milk

**Lunch**

Stir-fried vegetables (including mushrooms) in soy sauce

**Dinner**

Trout in Cider (page 178)
Mashed potatoes
Green beans
Carrots

Spiced Banana Parcels (page 184)

## Recipes

### Soups

#### Root Vegetable Soup

SERVES 4

3 tbsp sunflower oil
25 g (1 oz) margarine
1 medium onion, sliced
1 medium potato, chopped
1 medium parsnip, chopped
½ medium swede, chopped
2 small turnips, chopped
1 large carrot, chopped
900 ml (1½ pints) boiling water
1 level tbsp cornflour (less may be required)
black pepper to taste
1 tbsp soy sauce *or* 1 tsp yeast extract
coriander to garnish

Heat the oil and margarine and fry the vegetables for 1 minute stirring well. Add the water carefully. Bring back to the boil, then simmer in a covered pan for 3-4 minutes. Stir in the cornflour and black pepper, blended with a little cold water. Liquidize the vegetable mixture. Pour back into the pan and boil to thicken. Stir in the soy sauce (or yeast extract). Season to taste. Serve in bowls and garnish with coriander.

### Main courses

#### Chicken Korma

SERVES 4

3 tbsp vegetable oil
750 g (1½ lb) chicken, cubed
1 onion, chopped
1 clove garlic, crushed
1 tbsp each cumin and coriander
½ tsp each mild wheat-free curry powder and ginger
300 ml (½ pint) Greek yoghurt
2 tbsp desiccated coconut
300 ml (½ pint) chicken stock
50 g (2 oz) raisins
25 g (1 oz) flaked almonds
coriander sprigs to decorate

Heat the oil and cook the chicken until it is brown all over; remove and set aside. Gently cook the onion and garlic in the remaining oil for 2-3 minutes or until softened. Stir in the spices and yoghurt and cook for 2 minutes. Heat the stock, add the coconut and allow to stand for 2 minutes. Add both stock and chicken to the yoghurt mixture. Cover and simmer for 30 minutes until tender. Serve sprinkled with raisins, almonds and coriander.

## Blue Chicken Salad

### SERVES 2

175 g (6 oz) cooked skinned chicken, diced
50 g (2 oz) brown rice, cooked
50 g (2 oz) blue Cheshire cheese, cubed
1 eating apple, diced
25 g (1 oz) radish, sliced
1 stick celery, diced
15 g (½ oz) sultanas
3 tbsp natural yoghurt
1 red apple, sliced

Combine the chicken, rice, cheese, diced apple, radish, celery and sultanas. Fold the yoghurt into the mixture. Serve garnished with the red apple.

## Pork Chasseur

### SERVES 4

2 tsp oil
4 pork chops
1 onion, sliced
1 red pepper, sliced
100 g (4 oz) button mushrooms, sliced
1 tsp paprika
freshly ground black pepper
1 (400 g/14 oz) can chopped tomatoes
300 ml (½ pint) vegetable stock

Heat the oil in a large frying pan and brown the chops on both sides. Remove and keep warm. Add the onion to the pan and fry until soft but not brown, then stir in the red pepper, mushrooms and paprika. Season with black pepper. Continue frying for a further 5 minutes before adding the tomatoes and stock. Return the chops to the pan, cover and simmer gently for 45 minutes or until tender. Serve with potatoes and green vegetables.

## Trout in Cider

SERVES 2

2 small dessert apples, peeled and chopped
1 small onion, chopped
1 tbsp parsley, finely chopped
2 × 150-175 g (5-6 oz) trout, gutted
300 ml (½ pint) dry cider
freshly ground black pepper
2 lemon slices to garnish

Mix the apple and onion together with the parsley. Divide the mixture into two and use to stuff each trout.

Place the stuffed trout in an ovenproof dish. Pour the cider over and season with the pepper. Cover and cook in a preheated oven at Gas Mark 5 (190°C, 375°F) for 30-40 minutes. Serve with 2 tablespoons of the liquid spooned over each trout and a slice of lemon to garnish.

## Japanese Sardines

SERVES 4

10 ml (4 fl oz) wheat-free tamari
50 ml (2 fl oz) vinegar
2 tbsp lemon juice
25 g (1 oz) fresh root ginger, peeled and chopped
2 garlic cloves, crushed
450 g (1 lb) fresh sardines, washed thoroughly in cold water and dried

In a small mixing bowl, combine the wheat-free tamari, vinegar, lemon juice, ginger and garlic.

Arrange the sardines in a shallow baking dish and pour the soy sauce mixture over them. Leave in a cool place to marinate for 1½-2 hours.

Remove the sardines from the marinade and discard the marinade. Grill for 3-5 minutes or longer, depending on the size of the sardines, turning once. Serve immediately.

# Special Fried Rice

### SERVES 4

225 g (8 oz) long-grain rice
2 tsp sesame oil
1 egg, beaten
2 tbsp corn oil
1 onion, thinly sliced
1 clove garlic, crushed
100 g (4 oz) cooked chicken, diced
100 g (4 oz) peeled prawns
1 tbsp wheat-free tamari

Cook the rice according to the instructions on the packet, drain and rinse well. Heat the sesame oil in a small frying pan. Add the egg and let it cook into a type of omelette. Cut half of this into strips and chop the remaining half.

Heat the corn oil in a large frying pan. Add the onion and garlic and stir fry for 1 minute. Now add the rice, chicken, prawns and chopped omelette and stir fry for 4 minutes. Add the wheat-free tamari and stir fry well. Turn the mixture into a serving dish, arrange the omelette strips on top and serve. Serve with prawn crackers.

## Chinese Tuna Salad

SERVES 4

8 Chinese lettuce leaves, shredded
4 radishes, thinly sliced
1 bunch spring onions, finely chopped
1 medium cucumber, cut into matchsticks
50 g (2 oz) fresh bean-sprouts
4-8 canned water chestnuts, drained and thinly sliced
2 (200 g/7 oz) cans tuna in brine, drained and flaked

*Dressing*
1 tbsp wheat-free tamari
2 tbsp vegetable oil
1 tbsp fresh orange juice
1 tsp ground ginger
½ tsp caster sugar
freshly ground black pepper

Line a large serving dish (or 4 individual ones) with the lettuce leaves. Arrange the radish, spring onions, cucumber, bean-sprouts and chestnuts over the lettuce, then top with the tuna. In a jug, combine the dressing ingredients and blend together thoroughly with a fork. Serve the salad with the dressing separately.

## Steak Kebabs and Barbecue Sauce

SERVES 4

450 g (1 lb) steak, trimmed and cut into 2.5 cm (1 inch) cubes
8 small tomatoes
12 mushrooms, trimmed
1 onion
1 red pepper

*For the sauce*
5 tbsp lemon juice
5 tbsp wheat-free tamari
1 clove garlic, crushed
1 tsp finely chopped ginger
50 g (2 oz) polyunsaturated margarine

Thread the lamb, tomatoes, mushrooms, onion and pepper on to 4 long kebab skewers, alternating the ingredients. Combine all the sauce ingredients in a small pan and heat until the margarine has melted, stirring continuously. Heat the grill to Moderate and cook the kebabs for about 15 minutes, frequently basting them with the sauce. Serve with salad.

## Chicken Pilaff

SERVES 4

1 tbsp sunflower oil
4 bacon rashers, rinded and diced
1 onion, chopped
225 g (8 oz) long-grain rice
600 ml (1 pint) chicken stock
freshly ground black pepper
1 bay leaf
50 g (2 oz) sultanas
25 g (1 oz) toasted almonds, chopped
350 g (12 oz) cooked chicken meat, skinned and cubed

Pour the sunflower oil into a large saucepan, add the onion and bacon, and fry gently for 5 minutes until softened. Stir in the rice and stock and season with black pepper. Add the bay leaf and bring to the boil. Cover and simmer gently for 20 minutes until the rice is tender and all the liquid has been absorbed. Add the sultanas, almonds and chicken and cook gently, uncovered, for a further 5 minutes. Serve immediately.

## Stuffed Marrow

### SERVES 4-6

1 medium onion, chopped
1 clove garlic, crushed
175 g (6 oz) rice
100 g (4 oz) polyunsaturated margarine
100 g (4 oz) mushrooms, chopped
450 ml (¾ pint) hot water
1 tsp yeast extract
2 tsp dried mixed herbs
100 g (4 oz) nutmeat, diced
1 egg, beaten
1.5-1.75 kg (3-4 lb) marrow
chopped parsley or chives to decorate

Fry the onion, garlic and rice in 50 g (2 oz) margarine over low heat for 5 minutes. Stir in the mushrooms. Add the hot water, yeast extract and herbs. Cover and simmer until the water is absorbed – the rice doesn't need to be fully cooked. Stir in the nutmeat and egg and allow to cool.

Split the marrow lengthways and scoop out the seeds. Pile the stuffing into the centre. Brush the marrow shells with the remaining margarine, melted. Pack into a shallow ovenproof dish with 2-3 tbsp water and cover with foil. Cook on the top shelf of the oven at Gas Mark 4 (180°C, 350°F) for 40 minutes, by which time the top of the marrow should be browned. Sprinkle with parsley or chives to garnish.

## Mushroom Omelette

### SERVES 4

75 g (3 oz) margarine
350 g (12 oz) button mushrooms, thinly sliced
freshly ground black pepper
8 medium eggs
4 tbsp freshly chopped parsley
100 g (4 oz) vegetarian Cheddar cheese

Melt 25 g (1 oz) of the margarine in a saucepan. When the foam subsides, stir in the mushrooms and season with pepper. Cook gently for 3 minutes. Remove from the heat and keep warm.

For each omelette, break 2 eggs into a bowl and add 1 tbsp of parsley and seasoning. Beat lightly with a fork to mix. Melt a quarter of the remaining margarine in an omelette pan and set over a high heat. When the foam subsides, pour in the beaten eggs and stir the mixture with a fork. When the omelette is just set, spoon ¼ of the mushrooms and ¼ of the cheese on to one side. Fold over one half of the omelette on to the other to make an envelope. Keep it warm while making the remaining omelettes in the same way.

## *Desserts*

### Apricot Cake

MAKES ONE 23 CM (9 INCH) CAKE

225 g (8 oz) dried apricots
100 g (4 oz) hazelnuts
175 g (6 oz) caster sugar
6 eggs

Preheat the oven to Gas Mark 3 (160°C, 325°F). Put the apricots in a saucepan with 150 ml (¼ pint) of water. Simmer for a few minutes until they soften, then drain. Finely chop the hazelnuts. Blend the slightly cooled apricots to a paste and mix them in a bowl with the nuts and sugar. Separate the eggs and add the yolks to the mixture. Beat the whites and fold gradually into the mixture. Pour the mixture into a greased and floured 23 cm (9 inch) cake tin and bake for 1 hour. Cool in the tin before turning out.

## Pears with Port and Orange Sauce

### SERVES 4

200 ml (⅓ pint) port or red wine
1 tbsp grated orange rind
120 ml (4 fl oz) orange juice
120 ml (4 fl oz) water
6 tbsp caster sugar
4 ripe firm pears

Place the port (or wine), rind, juice and water in a large saucepan.
Bring to the boil, then add the sugar and stir until dissolved. Carefully peel the pears leaving the stalks intact. Add to the pan and turn
to coat them in syrup.

Stand the pears upright and simmer gently, basting frequently
with the syrup, for about 10 minutes until they are tender but not
mushy. Arrange the pears on a serving dish. Boil the sauce rapidly
until reduced by half. Then pour it over the pears, leave to cool and
chill in the refrigerator until ready to serve.

## Spiced Banana Parcels

### SERVES 4

4 firm bananas
75 g (3 oz) polyunsaturated margarine
1 tsp ground cinnamon
freshly grated nutmeg
50 g (2 oz) sultanas

Preheat the oven to Gas Mark 6 (200°C, 400°F). Cut 4 pieces of foil
20 cm (8 inches) square.

Melt 25 g (1 oz) margarine in a small saucepan and use to brush the
foil. Peel the bananas and place each on to a piece of foil. Sprinkle
with cinnamon and grate over a little nutmeg. Scatter the sultanas
over the top and dot with the remaining margarine. Fold up the foil
and crimp the edges to seal. Put the parcels on to a baking sheet and
bake for 10 minutes.

## Pear Paradise

SERVES 4

150 ml (¼ pint) red wine
150 ml (¼ pint) water
100 g (4 oz) caster sugar
4 pears, peeled and stalks intact
1 tsp arrowroot, optional

Mix the wine, water and sugar in a saucepan and dissolve over a gentle heat. Then boil until syrupy, without stirring. Stand the pears stalks upwards in the pan. Cut a circle of greaseproof paper with holes in for the stalks and place it over the pears. Boil for 5 minutes, basting occasionally until the pears are just tender. Carefully remove the pears to a serving dish. If the syrup is thin, boil it again and then stir in the arrowroot mixed with a little cold water. Boil for about 1 minute, until thick and clear. Allow to cool. Pour over and around the pears and serve.

## Brandied Apricot Flambé

SERVES 2

8 apricots, halved and stoned
6 tbsp water
4 tbsp caster sugar
1 tsp arrowroot
2 tbsp brandy

Place the halved apricots and water in a saucepan and heat gently. As the apricots soften, sprinkle the sugar over them and simmer on a very low heat until cooked but still hard. Strain the apricots (reserving the juice) and place in an ovenproof dish.

Mix the arrowroot with a little of the juice, mix with the remaining juice and return to the heat. Bring to the boil stirring constantly. Pour the thickened syrup over the apricots. Simmer the apricots and syrup on a low heat. Meanwhile, warm the brandy in a small saucepan.

Remove the apricots from the heat, gently pour the brandy over and ignite. Serve immediately.

## Carrot Cake
MAKES 10 SLICES

4 eggs
225 g (8 oz) caster (superfine) sugar
grated rind of 1 lemon
50 g (2 oz) sultanas
225 g (8 oz) ground almonds
225 g (8 oz) carrots, finely grated
1½ tbsp rice flour
1 tsp wheat-free baking powder

Preheat the oven to Gas Mark 4 (180°C, 350°F).

Separate the egg whites and yolks. Place the yolks, sugar and lemon rind in a bowl or blender and beat together well. Add the sultanas, almonds and carrots to this mixture. Stir well.

Sift the flour and baking powder together then fold into the mixture.

In another bowl beat the egg whites until they are stiff, then fold them into the mixture.

Grease an oblong baking sheet 20 × 30 × 5 cm (8 × 12 × 2 inches). Spread the mixture out in the tray and bake for 45 minutes. Leave to cool on the sheet, then cut into slices.

## Dried Fruit Compôte
SERVES 2

100 g (4 oz) mixture of dried fruits (e.g. peaches, prunes, apples, apricots and pears)
100 ml (4 fl oz) orange juice
2 whole cloves
5 cm (2 inch) stick of cinnamon
zest and juice of half a lemon

Wash the fruit and place in a bowl with the orange juice, spices, lemon juice and zest. Leave to soak overnight.

Next day, if the juice has been absorbed, add 2 tbsp water. Then place the mixture in a saucepan and bring to the boil. Cover and simmer on a very low heat for 10-15 minutes. Transfer to a serving bowl, removing the cinnamon and cloves. Serve warm or leave to cool.

# Phase 6
# oats, barley and rye week

## _____ Fast options _____

### *Lunches*

Pilchards and salad
Mackerel and salad
Sardines and salad
Tuna and salad

Prawn and Rice Salad (page 117)
Rice salad with chicken
Rice salad with nuts

Avocado and salad

Chicken and salad
Ham and salad
Turkey and salad

Rye crackers spread with mashed banana or sugar-free jam
Rye crackers with cheese and salad
Rye bread (wheat-free)
Barley Soup (page 192)
Oat cakes with spreads or cheese
Jordan's Frusli bars
Flapjacks (page 194)
Oat Crunchy cereal with fresh fruit, nuts and yoghurt

### *Dinners*

Chicken with vegetables and rice
Lamb chops and vegetables
Steak and vegetables
Grilled plaice with vegetables and rice
Steamed salmon with vegetables and rice

Stir-fried vegetables and rice, with prawns, nuts or chicken
Tomato omelette with vegetables
Prawn and egg salad
Cold meat salad
Grilled fish, rice and salad

Barley Cup (page 236)
Barley Soup (page 192)
Oat Cakes
Flapjacks (page 194)
Fruit Crumble (page 195)
Nutty Fruit (page 197)

## *Drinks and snacks*

### Hot drinks

Bambu (page 236)
Barley Cup (page 236)
Caro (page 236)
Chicory
2 cups of coffee (if no diarrhoea)
Dandelion coffee (boiled root) or instant dandelion coffee (if not
    intolerant to lactose)
Herbal teas, including fruit teas
Rooibosch, Eleven O'clock tea (especially good for gut spasm)
2 cups of tea (if not constipated)

### Cold drinks

Avoid alcohol
Apple juice/Appletise
Bottled water (with or without gas)
Tonic water

### Snacks

Baked Apple (page 125) or pear
Coconut Rounds (page 125)
Flapjacks (page 194)
Fruit Crumble (page 195)
Fruit salad (without citrus fruit)
Fruit sorbet (see recipes, pages 126, 153 and 154)
Gooseberry Jelly
Non-citrus fruits

Nutty Fruit (page 197)
Rice cakes, with sugar-free jam or mashed banana or hazelnut or
  almond butter
Rice salad
Oat cakes and spreads
Oat Crunchy cereal
Rye pumpernickel with savoury fillings
Rye crackers with butter, mashed banana or sugar-free jam
Soya ice cream
Soya yoghurt

## Menus

### Day 1

#### Breakfast

Porridge oats with milk and fresh fruit
Rice bread (toasted) with butter and sugar-free jam

#### Lunch

Mackerel in tomato sauce
Apple and Nut Salad (page 123)
2 rye crackers with butter

#### Dinner

Greek Hotpot (page 193)
Rice
Salad

Flapjacks (page 194)

### Day 2

#### Breakfast

Oat Crunchy cereal
Chopped fresh fruit with milk

#### Lunch

Orange and Carrot Soup (page 192)
Green salad
2 rye crackers with butter

## Dinner

Haddock Florentine (page 194)
Mashed potatoes
Carrots

Date Slices (page 195)

## Day 3

## Breakfast

Kellogg's Commonsense
Chopped fresh fruit and milk
Rice bread (toasted) with butter and sugar-free jam

## Lunch

Prawn, egg, lettuce and mayonnaise open sandwich on
    pumpernickel bread

## Dinner

Goulash (page 193)
Greens
Jacket potato

Fruit Crumble (page 195)

## Day 4

## Breakfast

Porridge oats with milk and fresh fruit
Rice bread (toasted) with butter and sugar-free jam

## Lunch

Barley Soup (page 192)
2 rye crackers with butter

## Dinner

Baked Chicken Burgers (page 112)
Chips
Salad

Apricot Pie (page 197)

## *Day 5*

### Breakfast

Oat Crunchy cereal with fresh fruit and milk
Rice bread (toasted) with butter and sugar-free jam

### Lunch

Chicken drumstick
Coleslaw and green salad
2 rye crackers with butter

### Dinner

Vegetable Loaf with Mustard Sauce (page 122)
Roast potatoes
Parsnips
Onions
Swede

Parkin (page 196)

## *Day 6*

### Breakfast

Kellogg's Commonsense cereal with raisins and milk
Rice bread (toasted) with butter and sugar-free jam

### Lunch

Rare roast beef, dried onions, lettuce and mustard pickle open
   sandwich on pumpernickel bread

### Dinner

Stuffed Mackerel (page 119)
Spinach
Courgettes
Peas

Flapjacks (page 194)

## *Day 7*

### Breakfast

Porridge oats
Dried fruit and milk
Rice bread (toasted) with butter and sugar-free jam

## Lunch
Barley Soup (page 192)
2 rye crackers with butter

## Dinner
Chicken with Almonds (page 112)
Rice
Broccoli
Sweetcorn

Nutty Fruit (page 197)

_____ Recipes _____

### *Soups*

### Barley Soup
SERVES 4

1 marrow bone
1.75-2.25 litres (3-4 pints) water
75 g (3 oz) pearl barley
3 carrots, diced
2 potatoes, diced
2 leeks, sliced
freshly ground black pepper
50 g (2 oz) butter beans (optional)

Place the marrow bone in the water and bring to the boil. Skim, then add the pearl barley, vegetables, seasoning and butter beans (if used). Bring to the boil and simmer for 1½-2 hours.

### Orange and Carrot Soup
SERVES 2

275 g (10 oz) carrots, chopped
1 medium leek, thinly sliced
350 ml (12 fl oz) vegetable stock
pinch of thyme
75-100 ml (3-4 fl oz) orange juice
freshly ground black pepper to taste

Place the carrots, leek, vegetable stock and thyme in a saucepan, bring to the boil and simmer for 30 minutes. Purée the mixture in a blender or food processor. Return to the saucepan and add the orange juice. Season with pepper, and heat through before serving.

## *Main courses*

### Greek Hotpot

SERVES 4

1 large onion, chopped
40 g (1½ oz) vegetable oil
450 g (1 lb) raw minced beef
2 tbsp porridge oats
1 (425 g/15 oz) can tomatoes
2 tbsp horseradish sauce
freshly ground black pepper
1 kg (2 lb) potatoes, peeled, cooked and sliced

Fry the onion in 25 g (1 oz) oil. When it starts to brown, add the mince and cook until the meat is sealed. Stir in the oats, tomatoes, horseradish and plenty of seasoning, then pour half the mixture into an ovenproof dish. Cover the meat with half the sliced potatoes, then repeat the two layers again. Arrange the potatoes so they neatly overlap the top. Dot the surface with rest of the oil and bake for 1½ hours, or until the potatoes are golden brown, at Gas Mark 4 (180°C, 350°F).

### Goulash

SERVES 4

750 g (1½ lb) stewing beef, cut into cubes
25 g (1 oz) cornflour
1 tbsp oil
1 large onion, chopped
1 tsp paprika
50 g (2 oz) pearl barley
freshly ground black pepper
3-4 potatoes, cut into quarters
1 (400 g/14 oz) can chopped tomatoes

Preheat the oven to Gas Mark 4 (180°C, 350°F).

Roll cubed meat in the cornflour. Heat the oil in a frying pan and add the meat and onion. Cook until slightly brown.

Place in a casserole dish and add the paprika, pearl barley and enough water to cover the meat. Season with the pepper. Cook for 1½ hours. Remove from the oven, add the cubed potatoes and tomatoes and cook for a further 20 minutes.

## Haddock Florentine

### SERVES 2

2 × 150 g (5 oz) haddock portions
225 g (8 oz) frozen spinach, defrosted and drained
2 tbsp lemon juice
2 slices lemon to garnish

Place each haddock portion on a separate piece of foil. Cover each portion with half the spinach and 1 tablespoon of lemon juice, and wrap in the foil.

Bake in a preheated oven for 20-30 minutes at Gas Mark 5 (190°C, 375°F). Remove the foil. Garnish each haddock portion with a slice of lemon and serve.

## *Desserts*

### Flapjacks

#### MAKES 8 TRIANGLES

50 g (2 oz) polyunsaturated margarine
25 g (1 oz) demerara sugar
25 g (1 oz) golden syrup
100 g (4 oz) rolled oats
pinch of salt

Heat the margarine in a large saucepan and stir in the other ingredients. Press into an 18 cm (7 inch) greased and floured sandwich tin. Bake at Gas Mark 5 (190°C, 375°F) for 20 minutes. Mark into triangles while hot and remove from the tin before completely cold.

## Fruit Crumble

### SERVES 4

750 g (1½ lb) cooking apples, cored and chopped
25 g (1 oz) raisins
6 tbsp unsweetened orange juice

*For the topping*
75 g (3 oz) porridge oats
2 tbsp melted polyunsaturated margarine
50 g (2 oz) fresh or dried dates, finely chopped
½ tsp ground cinnamon
1 tbsp desiccated coconut
1 tbsp chopped mixed nuts

Preheat the oven to Gas Mark 5 (190°C, 375°F). Place the apple in a 1.2 litre (2 pint) pie dish with the raisins and juice. Stir all the topping ingredients together and sprinkle over the apple. Bake for 30-35 minutes until the apple is soft.

## Date Slices

### MAKES 8 SLICES

250 ml (8 fl oz) water
75 g (3 oz) brown sugar
350 g (12 oz) chopped fresh or dried dates
¼ tsp lemon juice
225 g (8 oz) margarine
175 g (6 oz) brown sugar
175 g (6 oz) rice flour
175 g (6 oz) cornflour
¼ tsp bicarbonate of soda
2 tbsp water
175 g (6 oz) porridge oats

Preheat the oven to Gas Mark 4 (180°C, 350°F). To make the date filling, put the water and sugar in a saucepan over a low heat until the sugar is dissolved. Bring to the boil, add the dates and simmer gently, stirring constantly for 4-5 minutes. Remove from the heat, stir in the lemon juice and cool.

To prepare the oats mixture, cream the margarine in a mixing bowl until soft. Add the sugar and beat thoroughly until well creamed. Sift the rice flour and cornflour into the bowl and stir well until evenly blended. Dissolve the bicarbonate of soda in the water, then add to the flour mixture, stirring well. Stir in the oats.

Lightly press half the oats mixture into the bottom of a greased shallow 23 cm (9 inch) square tin. Cover with the cooled date mixture and top with the remaining oats mixture. Press down well. Bake for 45 minutes until golden brown. Cool in the tin, cut into squares and serve.

## Parkin

### SERVES 10

150 g (5 oz) golden syrup
150 g (5 oz) black treacle
100 g (4 oz) polyunsaturated margarine
100 g (4 oz) brown sugar
225 g (8 oz) brown rice flour
225 g (8 oz) rolled oats
1 tsp ground ginger
½ tsp bicarbonate of soda
150 ml (¼ pint) milk

Preheat the oven to Gas Mark 4 (180°C, 350°F). Grease a 23 × 18 cm (9 × 7 inch) tin and line with greaseproof paper. Put the syrup, treacle, margarine and sugar into a small pan and heat gently until melted.

Meanwhile mix together the flour, oats and ginger. Make a well in the centre and pour in the melted mixture. Mix thoroughly. Dissolve the bicarbonate of soda in the milk, then add to the mixture and stir well until evenly blended. Turn into the prepared tin. Bake for 50-60 minutes or until slightly shrinking away from the edges of the tin. Turn out and cool on a wire rack.

## Apricot Pie

SERVES 8

450 g (1 lb) cooked apricots or 1 large can
1 small can condensed milk
100 g (4 oz) polyunsaturated margarine
125 g (5 oz) rice flour
100 g (3 oz) cornflour
50 g (2 oz) rolled oats
50 g (2 oz) brown sugar

Strain the apricots and keep a few for decoration. Liquidize the fruit to a smooth pulp and mix with the condensed milk. Rub the margarine into the rice flour and cornflour until the mixture resembles breadcrumbs. Add the oats and sugar.

Preheat the oven to Gas Mark 5 (190°C, 375°F). Grease a round 18 cm (7 inch) loose-bottomed sandwich tin and press two-thirds of the crumb mixture over the bottom and sides of the tin. Put the apricot filling into the lined tin and cover with the rest of the crumbs. Do not press down. Bake for 30-35 minutes until golden. Decorate with the reserved apricots, cut into halves.

## Nutty Fruit

SERVES 4

750 g (1½ lb) mixed fruit (cherries, apples, blackberries, plums etc)
50 g (2 oz) brown rice flour
50 g (2 oz) porridge oats
1 tsp mixed spice
50 g (2 oz) polyunsaturated margarine
50 g (2 oz) brown sugar
25 g (1 oz) walnuts, chopped

Preheat the oven to Gas Mark 4 (180°C, 350°F). Prepare the fruit and place in an ovenproof dish. Mix together the flour, oats and mixed spice and rub in the margarine. Stir in the sugar and nuts and spoon over the fruit. Bake for 25-30 minutes until the fruit is tender and the topping golden.

# Phase 7
# white flour week

Tessa Lord is a 37-year-old health visitor. She has two children and lives with her husband in Salisbury. She contacted the WNAS for help in January 1993 after suffering with constipation all her life.

'I had been suffering with constipation, abdominal bloating and wind for as long as I can remember. The worst problem that this caused in latter years was haemorrhoids as a result of all the straining. I didn't consult my doctor about the problem as I wasn't keen to take laxatives in the long term.

'I enrolled on the WNAS postal and telephone course and a diet was designed to suit my needs. Within two months my symptoms were gone. In the main I stopped eating wheat products, took Linusit Gold with my cereal in the morning, and ate more vegetables and salad every day. I tried eating wheat again, but found that within 24 hours I had severe wind. I now open my bowels every morning routinely and am grateful for the help and advice I have received.'

## _____ Fast options _____

### *Lunches*

Pilchards and salad
Mackerel and salad
Sardines and salad
Tuna and salad

Prawn and Rice Salad (page 117)
Rice salad with chicken
Rice salad with nuts

Avocado and salad

Chicken and salad
Ham and salad
Turkey and salad

Quiche with salad
Scrambled egg on toast
Toasted sandwiches (using white bread)
White bread sandwiches
White rolls or fresh bread with fillings

## *Dinners*

Chicken with vegetables and rice
Lamb chops and vegetables
Steak and vegetables
Grilled plaice with vegetables and rice
Steamed salmon with vegetables and rice
Stir-fried vegetables and rice, with prawns, nuts or chicken
Tomato omelette with vegetables
Prawn and egg salad
Cold meat salad
Grilled fish, rice and salad
Steak-and-kidney pie (home-made)
Vegetable pie (home-made)
Beefburgers and buns
Sausages
Fried fish and chips
Lasagne (white flour)
Pizza
Fruit Crumble (page 195)
Apple pie
Danish pastry
Semolina
Shortbread (page 212)

## *Drinks and snacks*

### Hot drinks

Chicory
2 cups of coffee (if no diarrhoea)
Dandelion coffee (boiled root) or instant dandelion coffee (if not
    intolerant to lactose)

Herbal teas, including fruit teas
Rooibosch, Eleven O'clock Tea (especially good for gut spasm)
2 cups of tea (if not constipated)

## Cold drinks

Avoid alcohol
Apple juice/Appletise
Bottled water (with or without gas)
Tonic water

## Snacks

Baked Apple (page 125) or pear
Carrot and Walnut Squares (page 212)
Coconut Rounds (page 125)
Crumpets and scones
Fruit Crumble (page 195)
Fruit salad (without citrus fruit)
Fruit Sorbet (see recipes, pages 126, 153 and 154)
Gooseberry Jelly
Non-citrus fruits
Quiche
Rice cakes, with sugar-free jam or mashed banana or hazelnut or
    almond butter
Rice salad
Shortbread (page 212)
Soya ice cream
Soya yoghurt
White bread sandwiches or toast
White pasta salad

# Menus

## *Day 1*

## Breakfast
2 poached eggs and tomato on white toast

## Lunch
Courgette and Tomato Quiche (page 208)
Coleslaw
Apple and Nut Salad (page 123)

## Dinner

Spaghetti Bolognese
White pasta
Broccoli
Salad

Carrot and Walnut Squares (page 212)

## *Day 2*

## Breakfast

Cornflakes, fruit and nuts
White bread (toasted) with butter and sugar-free jam

## Lunch

Toasted cheese and tomato sandwich (white bread)
Mixed salad

## Dinner

Chicken and Sweetcorn Bake (page 204)
Mashed potatoes
Carrots
Peas

Apple Crumble (page 210)

## *Day 3*

## Breakfast

Toasted scrambled egg sandwich

## Lunch

Tuna Cakes (page 206)
Potato salad
Beansprout salad

## Dinner

Roast Beef in Garlic Crust (page 205)
Cauliflower
Roast potatoes
Carrots

Shortbread (page 212) and fruit salad

## *Day 4*

### Breakfast
Yoghurt with chopped fruit and nuts
White toast and sugar-free jam

### Lunch
Scotch Broth (page 204)
Chicken salad sandwich (white bread)

### Dinner
Fish Crumble (page 206)
Cauliflower
Courgettes

Semolina and sugar-free jam

## *Day 5*

### Breakfast
Rice Krispies
Chopped fruit and nuts
White toast and sugar-free jam

### Lunch
Toasted bacon, lettuce and tomato sandwich (white bread)
Walnut, Date and Marmalade Loaf (page 213)

### Dinner
Indian Meatballs in Tomato Sauce (page 207)
Pasta shells
Cauliflower

Bread and Butter Pudding (page 211)

## *Day 6*

### Breakfast
Poached egg and tomato with 2 rounds of white toast

### Lunch
Chicken and Sweetcorn Bake (page 204)
Ginger Biscuits (page 213)

## Dinner

Fried fish (in batter)
Chips
Peas
Salad

Lemon Fruit Roll (page 214)

## *Day 7*

## Breakfast

Pancakes spread with sugar-free jam
Fresh fruit salad

## Lunch

Stuffed Peppers (page 209)
Fresh fruit

## Dinner

Lasagne
Tomato and onion salad
Broccoli

Peach Cobbler (page 210)

# Recipes

## *Main courses*

### Scotch Broth

SERVES 4

50 g (2 oz) polyunsaturated margarine
1 small onion, finely chopped
1 small carrot, diced
1 small swede, diced
1 small parsnip, diced
1 small turnip, diced
1 small potato, diced
1 small leek, diced
50 g (2 oz) plain flour
1.5 litres (2½ pints) vegetable stock
100 g (4 oz) barley, cooked
freshly ground black pepper
1 small cauliflower, florets only, blanched

Heat the margarine in a deep pan. Add all the root vegetables and stir fry until the onions start to soften. Sprinkle flour over the mixture and stir in thoroughly. Allow to cool. Bring the stock to the boil and pour gradually over the vegetables stirring continuously.

Stir in the barley and season with pepper. Re-boil and add the cauliflower just before serving.

### Chicken and Sweetcorn Bake

SERVES 2

175 g (6 oz) onion, chopped
175 g (6 oz) red pepper, diced
175 g (6 oz) canned sweetcorn
2 tbsp water
175 g (6 oz) cooked chicken, diced
15 g (½ oz) plain flour
175 ml (6 fl oz) soya milk
freshly ground black pepper
1 tsp dried mixed herbs
75 g (3 oz) cheese, grated
75 g (3 oz) fresh white breadcrumbs

Preheat the oven to Gas Mark 4 (180°C, 350°F).

Combine the onions, red pepper and sweetcorn with the water. Simmer for 10 minutes and drain. Make a sauce with the flour, milk and black pepper. Combine the drained vegetables, chicken, sauce and herbs and pour into a casserole dish. Mix the cheese and breadcrumbs together and press on to the vegetable mixture. Bake for 15-20 minutes until brown.

## Roast Beef in Garlic Crust

SERVES 4

2.25 kg (5 lb) rib of beef
3 tbsp olive oil
3 cloves garlic, crushed
100 g (4 oz) fresh white breadcrumbs
3 tbsp chopped fresh parsley
½ tsp dried mixed herbs
1 tsp freshly ground black pepper

Preheat the oven to Gas Mark 4 (180°C, 350°F). Wipe the meat and place on a roasting rack. Heat the oil in a frying pan. Add the garlic and fry gently for 2 minutes stirring all the time. Mix in the breadcrumbs, parsley, herbs and pepper. Press the mixture on to the meat, coating well.

Roast the meat: 18-20 minutes per half kilo or pound for rare, 20-22 minutes for medium and 22-24 minutes for well done. Add a final extra 20 minutes. When cooked, remove, cover with foil and stand for 20 minutes before carving.

## Tuna Cakes

SERVES 4

1 (200 g/7 oz) can tuna in brine (drained)
350 g (12 oz) mashed potato˙
1 egg, beaten
2 tsp dried mixed herbs
½ tsp ground nutmeg
freshly ground black pepper
2 tbsp soya milk
4 tsp plain flour
2 tbsp olive oil

Flake the tuna into a bowl, add the potato, egg, herbs, nutmeg, pepper and milk. Mix thoroughly and form into 8 cakes. Dip fishcakes into the flour and fry in hot oil until crisp and golden brown. Drain and serve with salad.

## Fish Crumble

SERVES 2

1 clove garlic, finely chopped
1 small onion, thinly sliced
1 carrot, sliced
75 g (3 oz) green beans, sliced
½ tsp basil
1 tsp fresh chopped parsley
3 fresh tomatoes, peeled and sliced
200 g (7 oz) cod fillet
freshly ground black pepper
1 tbsp cornflour
1 tbsp water

*For the crumble*
50 g (2 oz) plain white flour
4 tsp polyunsaturated margarine

Place the garlic, onion, carrot, beans, basil, parsley and tomatoes in a saucepan.

Remove the skin from the fish and cut the fish into strips, about 4 cm (1½ inches) across. Add to the saucepan and season with pepper. Bring this mixture to the boil, cover, and reduce the heat. Simmer for 12-15 minutes.

Blend the cornflour to a paste with the water. Stir into the fish mixture and bring to the boil. Transfer the mixture to a deep, oven-proof dish.

To make the crumble topping, rub the flour and the margarine together until the mixture resembles breadcrumbs. Sprinkle the crumble over the fish and bake for 20-25 minutes at Gas Mark 4 (180°C, 350°F).

## Indian Meatballs in Tomato Sauce

### SERVES 4

450 g (1 lb) minced lamb
50 g (2 oz) fresh white breadcrumbs
1 egg
1 tsp ground coriander
1 tsp mild chilli powder
½ tsp cumin seed
½ tsp turmeric
1 clove garlic, crushed
1 onion, finely chopped
½ tsp black pepper
2 tbsp oil
1 (400 g/14 oz) can tomatoes
coriander to garnish

Mix together the lamb, breadcrumbs, egg, spices, garlic, onion and pepper. Divide the mixture into 24 small meatballs using wetted hands. Heat the oil in a large frying pan and fry gently until browned all over. Add the tomatoes and simmer for a further 15 minutes until the meatballs are cooked through. Serve garnished with coriander.

## Courgette and Tomato Gratin

SERVES 4

1 kg (2 lb) courgettes
75 g (3 oz) polyunsaturated margarine
1 small clove garlic, crushed
2 tbsp chopped parsley
450 g (1 lb) tomatoes, skinned and chopped
freshly ground black pepper
50 g (2 oz) fresh white breadcrumbs

Trim the courgettes and slice into rounds 5 mm (¼ inch) thick. Preheat the oven to Gas Mark 7 (220°C, 425°F). Melt 15 g (½ oz) margarine in a saucepan and add the garlic, parsley, tomatoes and pepper. Let the tomatoes cook gently for about 15 minutes, until reduced to a thick purée, but not too dry. Remove from the heat and leave to one side.

Rinse the courgettes and pat dry. Melt 25 g (1 oz) margarine in a large saucepan. Add half the courgette slices and fry gently until soft and transparent, not brown. Remove and set aside. Repeat with the rest of the courgettes. Gently mix the courgettes with the tomato sauce. Adjust seasoning if required. Spoon the mixture into a shallow casserole dish and smooth the top. Sprinkle with the breadcrumbs and dot with the remaining 15 g (½ oz) margarine. Bake in the oven for 25-30 minutes until golden brown and bubbling.

## Courgette and Tomato Quiche

SERVES 4-6

225 g (8 oz) shortcrust pastry
50 g (2 oz) polyunsaturated margarine
2 garlic cloves, crushed
4 courgettes, trimmed and sliced
freshly ground black pepper to taste
½ tsp oregano
100 ml (4 fl oz) milk
3 eggs
50 g (2 oz) Cheddar cheese, grated
5 small tomatoes, peeled and thinly sliced

Line a flan dish with the pastry and set aside.

Preheat the oven to Gas Mark 6 (200°C, 400°F).

Melt the margarine in a large frying pan. Add the garlic and fry, stirring frequently for 1 minute. Add the courgettes and pepper. Fry for 8-10 minutes or until lightly browned. Remove the pan from the heat and add the oregano, mixing well to blend.

In a mixing bowl combine the milk, eggs and cheese. Beat well to blend.

Arrange the courgettes and tomatoes in circles in the pastry flan case. Pour the egg, milk and cheese mixture over the courgettes and tomatoes. Place in the centre of the oven and bake for 35-45 minutes or until the filling is set and golden brown.

## Stuffed Peppers

SERVES 4

4 medium peppers
freshly ground black pepper
275 g (10 oz) lean minced beef
1 medium onion, chopped
50 g (2 oz) mushrooms
50 g (2 oz) tomatoes
1 slice white bread toasted and cubed
2 tbsp beef stock
½ tsp wholegrain mustard

Preheat the oven to Gas Mark 4 (180°C, 350°F). Cut off and reserve the tops of the peppers to use as lids. Core and seed the peppers, then cook for 5 minutes in a large saucepan of boiling water. Drain and season well inside.

Place beef and onion in a non-stick frying pan and fry without adding fat. Stir until evenly browned. Stir in the mushrooms, tomatoes, bread, stock and mustard and season to taste. Spoon the mixture into the peppers and replace the tops. Place upright in a baking dish and bake for 25 minutes until tender. Serve hot with rice or cold with salad. You can use minced pork or finely chopped chicken as an alternative to beef.

## *Desserts*

### Apple Crumble

SERVES 6

*For the topping*
100 g (4 oz) plain flour, sifted
100 g (4 oz) caster sugar
75 g (3 oz) polyunsaturated margarine

*For the filling*
1 kg (2 lb) cooking apples, peeled, cored and quartered
1 tsp ground cinnamon
50 g (2 oz) caster sugar
4 tbsp lemon juice
4 tbsp water

Preheat the oven to Gas Mark 5 (190°C, 375°F). To make the topping, mix the flour and sugar and then stir in the margarine. Rub in lightly until evenly mixed. To make the filling, slice the apples and put them into a buttered pie dish. Mix the cinnamon with the sugar and sprinkle over. Mix lemon juice and water and pour over. Spread the crumble topping evenly over the apples so that the dish is completely sealed. Bake for 40 minutes until golden brown.

### Peach Cobbler

SERVES 4

6-8 fresh peaches
100 g (4 oz) sugar
1 tbsp cornflour
finely grated rind of lemon
1 tbsp lemon juice
few drops almond essence
1 tbsp polyunsaturated margarine

*For the topping*
175 g (6 oz) self-raising flour
25 g (1 oz) sugar
90 g (3½ oz) polyunsaturated margarine
120 ml (4 fl oz) milk
1 egg, beaten
1 tsp caster sugar
2 tsp cinnamon

Peel and slice the peaches. Mix the sugar, cornflour and lemon rind. Add the peaches and fold together. Sprinkle with lemon juice and almond essence. Empty into a greased, large shallow ovenproof dish. Cook in a preheated oven at Gas Mark 4 (180°C, 350°F) for about 15 minutes, until hot and bubbling.

Prepare the topping while the peaches are cooking. Sift the flour and sugar, and rub in the margarine lightly. Add the milk to the beaten egg and mix with the flour and margarine mixture, making a dough. Roll into small scones and place on top of the peaches. Sprinkle the caster sugar and cinnamon over and bake for a further 30 minutes until golden.

## Bread and Butter Pudding

SERVES 4

8 slices white bread, well buttered, crusts removed
grated rind of 1 orange
50 g (2 oz) brown sugar
50 g (2 oz) sultanas
300 ml (½ pint) milk
1 egg
¼ tsp vanilla essence

Grease a 900 ml (1½ pint) pie dish with butter. Cut the bread slices into 3 and arrange half the bread buttered-side down in the dish. Cover with half the orange rind, half the sugar and the sultanas. Cover with the remaining bread. Sprinkle with the remaining dry ingredients. Mix the milk, egg and essence together, and pour over the pudding. Leave to soak for 30 minutes. Bake in the centre of a preheated oven at Gas Mark 4 (180°C, 350°F) for 45-50 minutes until golden brown.

## Carrot and Walnut Squares

MAKES 8 SQUARES

275 g (10 oz) plain flour
1 tsp bicarbonate of soda
2 tsp baking powder
175 g (6 oz) caster sugar
175 g (6 oz) carrots, grated
50 g (2 oz) walnut pieces
2 small bananas, mashed
175 ml (6 fl oz) sunflower oil
3 eggs

*For the frosting*
50 g (2 oz) butter
100 g (4 oz) icing sugar, sifted
50 g (2 oz) full fat soft cheese
few drops vanilla essence
walnuts to decorate

Grease and line the base of an 18 × 28cm (7 × 11 inch) baking tin with greaseproof paper. In a bowl, mix the flour, bicarbonate of soda and baking powder. Add the sugar, carrots, nuts and bananas. Beat the oil and eggs together. Pour on to the mixture and mix well. Spoon into the baking tin and level the surface. Bake in a preheated oven at Gas Mark 4 (180°C, 350°F) for 30-35 minutes until the cake is well risen. Cool in the tin for 10 minutes, then turn out and remove the paper. Leave to cool.

To make the frosting, beat the butter and icing sugar until fluffy. Stir in the cheese and vanilla essence and spread over the cake. Decorate with walnuts.

## Shortbread

MAKES 10-12 PIECES

100 g (4 oz) polyunsaturated margarine
50 g (2 oz) caster sugar
150 g (5 oz) plain flour
25 g (1 oz) semolina
extra sugar to sprinkle over the top

Cream together the fat and the sugar. Gradually stir in the flour and semolina, using a fork. Bind the mixture together well and press into an 18 cm (7 inch) circular tin lined with greaseproof paper. Prick very well with a fork. Bake in a preheated oven at Gas Mark 4 (180°C, 350°F) for 10-15 minutes until golden brown. Leave to cool in the tin, remove and sprinkle over a little extra sugar. Leave to go cold before serving.

## Ginger Biscuits

### MAKES 12 BISCUITS

225 g (8 oz) plain flour
2 tsp ground ginger
150 g (5 oz) demerara sugar
100 g (4 oz) cooking Flora
1 large egg
1 level tsp bicarbonate of soda
1 tbsp soya milk

Sift together the flour, ginger and sugar. Rub in the fat and add the egg and bicarbonate of soda dissolved in the milk. Mix well and knead on a floured board, taking care not to let the mixture become too stiff. Form into balls, place on a greased baking tray and flatten a little.

Bake in a preheated oven for 30 minutes at Gas Mark 3 (160°C, 325°F). Allow to cool. You can also make these biscuits using self-raising flour, in which case omit the bicarbonate of soda.

## Walnut, Date and Marmalade Loaf

### SERVES 6-8

100 g (4 oz) dates, chopped
65 ml (2½ fl oz) water
40 g (1½ oz) polyunsaturated margarine
1 tbsp marmalade
175 g (6 oz) self-raising flour
1 tbsp milk
1 egg, beaten
50 g (2 oz) walnuts, chopped

Preheat the oven to Gas Mark 4 (180°C, 350°F). Place the dates, water, margarine and marmalade in a small saucepan. Bring to the boil, then simmer for 2 minutes. Allow to cool. In a bowl, mix together the flour, milk, egg and walnuts. When thoroughly mixed, add the date and marmalade mixture and combine thoroughly. Put into a greased and lined 450 g (1 lb) baking tin and bake for 50-55 minutes until risen and a skewer comes out clean.

## Lemon Fruit Roll

MAKES APPROXIMATELY 10 SLICES

½ tsp sunflower oil
3 eggs
grated rind of 1 lemon
1 level tbsp concentrated apple juice
50 g (2 oz) white self-raising flour
2 tbsp hot water
4 tbsp lemon curd
4 rings canned pineapple in natural juice, chopped

Line a swiss roll tin (20 × 28 cm/8 × 11 inches) with greaseproof paper and brush lightly with the oil.

Separate the eggs and whisk the yolks together with the grated lemon rind and the concentrated apple juice until light and creamy.

Sieve the flour and fold into the egg mixture together with the water.

Whisk the egg whites until stiff and then fold gently into the mixture. Gently place the mixture in the prepared swiss roll tin and bake in a preheated oven for 12-15 minutes at Gas Mark 6 (200°C, 400°F).

Turn out on to a sheet of greaseproof paper and trim the edges. Roll up with the paper inside and leave to cool. Unroll the swiss roll gently, and spread with the lemon curd and chopped pineapple pieces. Roll up again and place on a serving dish.

# Phase 8
# wholewheat week

## Fast options

### *Lunches*

Pilchards and salad
Mackerel and salad
Sardines and salad
Tuna and salad

Prawn and Rice Salad (page 117)
Rice salad with chicken
Rice salad with nuts

Avocado and salad

Chicken and salad
Ham and salad
Turkey and salad

Muesli with fresh fruit
Scrambled egg on wholemeal toast
Toasted (wholemeal bread) sandwiches
Wholemeal and wholewheat bread rolls and buns
Wholemeal pasta and spaghetti
Wholemeal quiche with salad
Wholemeal rolls with fillings
Wholemeal sandwiches

### *Dinners*

Chicken with vegetables and rice
Lamb chops and vegetables
Steak and vegetables
Grilled plaice with vegetables and rice
Steamed salmon with vegetables and rice

Stir-fried vegetables and rice, with prawns, nuts or chicken
Tomato omelette with vegetables
Prawn and egg salad
Cold meat salad
Grilled fish, rice and salad
Steak-and-kidney pie (home-made)
Vegetable pie (home-made)
Beefburgers and buns
Sausages
Fried fish and chips
Lasagne (wholemeal flour)
Pizza (wholemeal or wholewheat flour)
Wholemeal lasagne
Fruit Crumble (wholemeal or wholewheat flour) (page 195)
Apple tart (wholemeal or wholewheat flour) (page 228)
Danish pastry (wholemeal or wholewheat flour)
Semolina
Shortbread (wholemeal or wholewheat flour) (page 212)
Wholemeal Pancakes (page 223)
Shredded wheat with banana and milk
Carrot Cake (page 186)

## *Drinks and snacks*

### Hot drinks

Chicory
2 cups of coffee (if no diarrhoea)
Dandelion coffee (boiled root) or instant dandelion coffee (if not
    intolerant to lactose)
Herbal teas, including fruit teas
Rooibosch, Eleven O'clock tea (especially good for gut spasm)
2 cups of tea (if not constipated)

### Cold drinks

Avoid alcohol
Apple juice/Appletise
Bottled water (with or without gas)
Tonic water

## Snacks

Apple Tart (page 228)
Baked Apple (page 125) or pear
Coconut Rounds (page 125)
Fruit salad (without citrus fruit)
Fruit sorbet (see pages 126, 153 and 154)
Gooseberry Jelly
Muesli
Non-citrus fruits
Rice cakes, with sugar-free jam or mashed banana or hazelnut or
    almond butter
Rice salad
Slice of pizza
Soya ice cream
Soya yoghurt
Wholemeal Pancakes (page 223)
Wholemeal toast or sandwich

# Menus

## *Day 1*

### Breakfast

Muesli and fresh fruit
Wholemeal toast and sugar-free jam

### Lunch

Pizza Toast (page 226)
Green salad
Wholemeal Date, Banana and Hazelnut Bread (page 226)

### Dinner

Chicken Pie (page 222)
Mashed potatoes
Sweetcorn
Green beans

Carrot and Date Cake (page 229)

## *Day 2*

### Breakfast
Wholemeal Pancakes (page 223) with mushrooms and tomatoes

### Lunch
Tuna and salad wholemeal sandwich

### Dinner
Fish Crumble (wholemeal flour) (page 206)
Carrots
Cauliflower
Cabbage

Mixed fruit tart

## *Day 3*

### Breakfast
Weetabix and milk
Wholewheat toast and sugar-free jam

### Lunch
Broccoli and sweetcorn
Quiche made with wholemeal pastry
Mixed salad

### Dinner
Turkey in Wholemeal Breadcrumbs (page 225)
Hot potato salad
Peas
Carrots

Apple and blackberry pie

## *Day 4*

### Breakfast
Shredded Wheat
Banana and milk
Wholemeal toast and sugar-free jam

**Lunch**

Prawn salad in wholemeal roll

**Dinner**

Wholewheat Spaghetti with Ham and Spinach Sauce (page 225)

Wholemeal Pancakes (page 223) with mixed fruit sauce

## *Day 5*

**Breakfast**

Muesli and fresh fruit
Wholemeal toast with sugar-free jam

**Lunch**

Cheese on wholemeal toast
Green salad

**Dinner**

Vegetable Macaroni Bake (page 221)
Mange-touts

Rhubarb Brownie (page 229)

## *Day 6*

**Breakfast**

Weetabix and fresh fruit
Wholemeal toast and sugar-free jam

**Lunch**

Winter Stew with Dumplings (page 220)

**Dinner**

Marinated Trout (page 223)
Boiled potatoes
Broccoli
Carrots

Fruit and Nut Crumble (page 227)

## Day 7

### Breakfast

Shredded Wheat and banana
Wholemeal toast and sugar-free jam

### Lunch

Egg and cress wholemeal sandwich
Wholemeal and Bran Muffins (page 227)

### Dinner

Curried Beef Wholemeal Pancakes (page 224)
Courgettes
Cauliflower
Mango chutney

Apple Tart (page 228)

## Recipes

### *Main courses*

#### Winter Stew with Dumplings

SERVES 4

2 tbsp vegetable oil
1 onion, chopped
2 carrots, sliced
175 g (6 oz) turnip, diced
1-2 parsnips, cut into short lengths
2 leeks, sliced
3 potatoes, cut into chunks
1 tsp plain white flour
1.2 litres (2 pints) hot vegetable stock
1 tbsp tomato purée
freshly ground black pepper
1 tbsp chopped fresh parsley

*For the dumplings*
175 g (6 oz) wholemeal self-raising flour
25 g (1 oz) polyunsaturated margarine
1 tsp dried mixed herbs
freshly ground black pepper to taste
1 tbsp vegetable oil
8 tbsp water

Heat a little of the oil in a pan and fry the onion quickly until golden brown. Transfer to a large casserole dish. Adding a little more oil each time, quickly brown each vegetable and then transfer into the casserole. When all the vegetables have been browned, add a little more oil, stir in the flour and cook over a steady heat, stirring all the time until the flour is browned. Pour in the hot stock and bring to the boil, stirring continuously until the stock has thickened slightly. Add the tomato purée and plenty of black pepper, then pour over the vegetables. Put a lid on the casserole and cook in the oven at Gas Mark 4 (180°C, 350°F) for 50 minutes.

Meanwhile make the dumplings. Put the flour into a bowl and rub in the margarine until the mixture resembles breadcrumbs. Add the herbs and season with the black pepper. Mix to a very soft dough with the oil and water. Turn on to a floured surface and divide into 8 pieces. Shape lightly into a ball. When the stew has cooked for 50 minutes add the dumplings, replace the lid and cook for a further 20-30 minutes. The dumplings will rise to the top and double in size. Sprinkle with parsley and serve immediately.

## Vegetable Macaroni Bake

### SERVES 4-6

100 g (4 oz) dried red kidney beans, soaked overnight
225 g (8 oz) wholewheat macaroni
freshly ground black pepper
25 g (1 oz) polyunsaturated margarine
25 g (1 oz) cornflour
300 ml (½ pint) milk
1 tbsp vegetable oil
1 leek sliced
1 courgette, sliced
350 g (12 oz) tomatoes, skinned and chopped
1-2 tsp dried basil
100 g (4 oz) Parmesan cheese, grated
2 slices wholemeal bread, crusts removed
100 g (4 oz) Cheddar cheese, grated

Drain the kidney beans, rinse and put into a saucepan with double the amount of water. Bring to the boil, cover and boil vigorously for 10 minutes. Lower the heat and simmer gently for 1 hour until tender. Drain well.

Meanwhile cook the macaroni in plenty of boiling water for 12 minutes, and drain thoroughly. Preheat the oven to Gas Mark 5 (190°C, 375°F). Melt the margarine in a saucepan, stir in the cornflour and then gradually stir in the milk. Cook stirring over a low heat until thickened. Season to taste.

Heat the oil in another pan, add the garlic, leek, carrot and courgette and fry gently for 5 minutes until softened. Add the tomatoes, basil and kidney beans, then stir into white sauce with the pasta and Parmesan cheese. Spoon into a greased shallowproof dish. Make breadcrumbs from the bread and mix with the Cheddar cheese. Sprinkle over the pasta mixture. Bake in the oven for 30-35 minutes. Serve hot.

## Chicken Pie

SERVES 6

25 g (1 oz) polyunsaturated margarine
25 g (1 oz) plain flour
150 ml (¼ pint) chicken stock
150 ml (¼ pint) milk
1 tsp curry powder
2 small carrots, sliced
750 g (1½ lb) cooked chicken, diced
100 g (4 oz) ham, diced
100 g (4 oz) frozen sweetcorn
100 g (4 oz) cooking Flora
225 g (8 oz) wholemeal flour
2 tbsp water

Preheat the oven to Gas Mark 6 (200°C, 400°F). Melt the margarine in a pan and stir in the flour until blended. Remove from the heat and gradually stir in the stock and milk. Return to the heat and bring to the boil, stirring constantly. Simmer for 2 minutes, season to taste, and stir in the curry powder. Add the carrots, chicken, ham and sweetcorn to the sauce and place in a 900 ml (1½ pint) pie dish.

Place the wholemeal flour in a bowl. Rub in the Flora until the mixture resembles breadcrumbs. Add water and mix to form a smooth dough. Allow to rest for 15 minutes. Roll out the pastry on a floured surface until it is large enough to fit the pie dish. Place over the top and trim neatly. Decorate with any trimmings and bake for 30 minutes until the pastry is golden brown.

## Marinated Trout

SERVES 4

2 tbsp olive oil
2 whole trout (225 g/8 oz each), cleaned
2 tbsp plain wholemeal flour
1 small fennel bulb, trimmed and finely sliced
1 medium onion, skinned and finely sliced
300 ml (½ pint) dry white wine
finely grated rind and juice of 1 orange
freshly ground black pepper
orange slices to garnish

Heat the oil in a frying pan. Dip each trout in the flour and fry gently for 4 minutes on each side. Transfer to a shallow dish when cooked. Score the skin diagonally but not too deeply into the flesh. Set aside. Add the fennel and onion to the pan and fry for 5 minutes. Add the wine, orange rind, juice and pepper to taste. Bring to the boil and boil rapidly for 1 minute. Pour immediately over the fish and cool. Marinate in the fridge for 8-12 hours. Serve at room temperature garnished with orange slices.

## Wholemeal Pancakes

SERVES 4

100 g (4 oz) wholemeal flour
1 small egg
300 ml (½ pint) skimmed milk
oil for cooking

Make a thin batter with the flour, egg and skimmed milk, whisking well.

Use kitchen paper to wipe a small non-stick frying pan with oil and heat until it is smoking.

Pour a generous 2 tablespoons of the batter into the pan and swirl it around to cover the bottom as thinly as possible. Cook the batter for 60 seconds, then flip it over with a spatula and cook the other side for a few seconds only. If you are going to eat straight away, tip on to a heated plate – otherwise stacked pancakes with cling film in between can be stored in the refrigerator. They can be easily reheated individually on a plate covered with foil over a pan of water or in the microwave oven.

## Curried Beef Wholemeal Pancakes
### SERVES 4

100 g (4 oz) plain wholemeal flour
1 egg
300 ml (½ pint) skimmed milk
1 tsp sunflower oil

*For the filling*
4 level tbsp skimmed milk powder
2 level tsp curry powder
2 level tbsp cornflour
600 ml (1 pint) water
2 level tbsp apricot jam
4 level tbsp mango chutney
2 tbsp WeightWatchers Beef Soup
freshly ground black pepper to taste
350 g (12 oz) minced beef
1 medium onion, finely chopped
2 tbsp tomato purée

Make a thin batter with the flour, egg and milk, whisking well. Heat the oil in a small frying pan. Pour a little of the batter into the pan and swirl it around to cover the bottom of the pan as thinly as possible. Cook for 60 seconds, then flip it over to cook the other side for a few seconds only. Continue like this with the remaining batter. (The mixture will make approximately 8 thin pancakes.)

To make the filling, mix the milk powder, half the curry powder and the cornflour with enough water to make a smooth paste. Mix with the remaining water and pour into a saucepan. Add to this the apricot jam, mango chutney and beef soup. Season with the pepper. Bring gently to the boil and simmer gently for 2 minutes. Put to one side.

Brown the mince in a frying pan. Strain off the excess fat and add the chopped onions, the remaining curry powder, the tomato purée and about one third of the curry sauce. Stir well. Simmer in covered pan for 15 minutes, stirring occasionally. Add a little water if necessary to prevent the mixture drying.

Fill each of the pancakes with the curry mixture and roll them up. Place them in a covered ovenproof dish and then into a preheated oven for 12 minutes at Gas Mark 5 (190°C, 375°F).

Heat the remaining curry sauce and pour a little over each pancake just before serving.

# Wholewheat Spaghetti with Ham and Spinach Sauce

### SERVES 4

1 medium onion, chopped
225 g (8 oz) frozen chopped spinach
300 ml (½ pint) boiling water
½ level tbsp mixed dried herbs
50 g (2 oz) skimmed milk powder
1 level tbsp cornflour
85 ml (3 fl oz) cold water
100 g (4 oz) wholewheat spaghetti
freshly ground black pepper to taste
175 g (6 oz) cooked lean ham, chopped into small pieces

Place the onion in a saucepan with the spinach, boiling water and mixed herbs. Cover the pan and simmer gently for 5 minutes.

Purée the onion and spinach mixture in a liquidizer or food processor.

Blend the skimmed milk powder and cornflour with the cold water. Place in the saucepan with the spinach purée, and bring to the boil, stirring constantly. Simmer for 1-2 minutes.

Meanwhile, boil the spaghetti for 12-15 minutes until just tender.

Add the ham to the sauce, season with freshly ground black pepper, and heat for 1-2 minutes.

To serve, drain the spaghetti and divide between four plates and top with the sauce.

# Turkey in Wholemeal Breadcrumbs

### SERVES 1

1 egg
100 g (4 oz) turkey breast
1 tbsp wholemeal breadcrumbs

Whisk the egg and brush over the turkey breast.

Place the breadcrumbs in a shallow bowl and dip the turkey breast on both sides until coated. Place the turkey breast on a sheet of foil, and grill for 15-20 minutes, turning occasionally, until cooked.

## Pizza Toast
SERVES 1

2 slices of wholemeal toast

*For the topping*
1 tsp oil
½ onion, chopped
1 small garlic clove, crushed
2 large tomatoes, skinned and chopped
½ tsp mixed herbs
1 tbsp tomato purée
¼ small green pepper, chopped
2 sardines, canned in tomato sauce, drained

Heat the oil in a frying pan and fry the onion and garlic for 2-3 minutes. Add the tomatoes, mixed herbs, tomato purée and chopped peppers and simmer for a further 2-3 minutes.

Chop the sardines and add to the sauce. Stir until the sardines are heated through.

Cover each slice of toast with the sauce. Place under a medium grill for 1 minute.

## *Desserts*

## Wholemeal Date, Banana and Hazelnut Bread
SERVES 10-12

225 g (8 oz) stoned dried dates, roughly chopped
1 tsp bicarbonate of soda
300 ml (½ pint) semi-skimmed milk
275 g (10 oz) self-raising wholemeal flour
100 g (4 oz) polyunsaturated margarine
75 g (3 oz) shelled hazelnuts, chopped
2 ripe bananas
1 egg, beaten
2 tbsp clear honey

Grease and line a 1 kg (2 lb) loaf tin. Put the dates in a pan with the bicarbonate of soda and milk. Bring slowly to boiling point, stirring, remove from the heat and leave until cold. Put the flour into a large bowl and rub in the margarine with fingertips. Stir in the hazelnuts, reserving 2 tbsp for decoration. Peel and mash the bananas, then add them to the flour mixture with the dates and egg. Beat well to mix. Spoon the mixture into the prepared tin. Bake in the oven at Gas Mark 4 (180°C, 350°F) for 1-1¼ hours until an inserted skewer comes out clean. Leave the loaf to cool in the tin for 5 minutes. Turn out, remove the lining paper and place the right way up on a cooling rack. Heat the honey gently, then brush over the top of the loaf. Sprinkle on the reserved hazelnuts and leave until cold.

## Wholemeal and Bran Muffins

### MAKES 4

65 g (3 oz) plain wholemeal flour
65 g (3 oz) bran
1½ tsp baking powder
1 egg, beaten
300 ml (½ pint) semi-skimmed milk
2 tbsp honey

Grease a 4 hole patty tin. Mix the flour, bran and baking powder together in bowl. Make a well in the centre and add the egg. Stir vigorously to mix, then add the milk and honey. Beat to a smooth batter. Pour the batter into the prepared tins. Bake in a preheated oven at Gas Mark 5 (190°C, 375°F) for 25 minutes until risen. Turn out on to a wire rack and cool for 5 minutes. Serve split in half and spread with margarine.

## Fruit and Nut Crumble

### SERVES 4

100 g (4 oz) plain wholemeal flour
50 g (2 oz) polyunsaturated margarine
100 g (4 oz) demerara sugar
25 g (1 oz) walnuts, finely chopped
3 cooking pears
1 large cooking apple
2 tbsp redcurrant jelly
finely grated rind and juice of 1 lemon

Place the flour and margarine in a bowl. Rub in until the mixture resembles breadcrumbs. Stir in half of the sugar and walnuts. Set aside. Peel and quarter the pears and apples. Remove the cores and slice the flesh thinly. In a bowl, mix together the redcurrant jelly, lemon rind, juice and remaining sugar. Add the sliced fruit and fold gently to mix. Turn the fruit into an ovenproof dish and sprinkle the crumble mixture over the top. Bake in a preheated oven at Gas Mark 4 (180°C, 350°F) for 40 minutes or until the fruit feels soft when pierced with a skewer and the topping is crisp and golden. Serve hot.

## Apple Tart

SERVES 8

*For the base*
100 g (4 oz) wholemeal flour
50 g (2 oz) butter, cut into pieces
50 g (2 oz) Cheddar cheese, grated

*For the filling*
450 g (1 lb) cooking apples, peeled, cored and sliced
150 ml (¼ pint) unsweetened orange juice
knob of butter
¼ tsp ground cloves

*To decorate*
1 large red dessert apple
1 large green dessert apple
300 ml (½ pint) unsweetened apple juice
1 tbsp apple concentrate

Preheat the oven to Gas Mark 6 (200°C, 400°F). Grease a 20 cm (8 inch) flan ring. To make the base, place the flour in a bowl, add the butter and rub in. Stir in the cheese and sufficient water to make a soft dough. Knead on a floured surface until smooth. Use to line the base and sides of flan ring. Prick and bake blind for 15-20 minutes until golden and base is dry. Leave to cool.

To make the filling, place all the filling ingredients into a saucepan, cover and cook over a low heat until the apples are soft. Beat until smooth. Cool and chill. Place the pastry case on a serving plate and spread the chilled apple purée over the base.

To decorate, wash, core and very thinly slice one dessert apple. Boil the apple juice in a large pan for 1 minute. Add half the prepared apple. Reduce the heat and simmer for 30 seconds. Remove the apple with a draining spoon and place on absorbent paper. Repeat with the remaining apple. Remove the pan from the heat. Arrange alternating slices of red and green apple over the apple purée. Stir the apple concentrate in the pan, boil until it is reduced by half and makes a coating consistency. Quickly brush over the apple slices to glaze. Chill the tart until required – though it is best eaten on the day it is made.

## Rhubarb Brownie

SERVES 4

450 g (1 lb) rhubarb
225 g (8 oz) fresh wholemeal breadcrumbs
50 g (2 oz) raw cane sugar
½ tsp ground ginger
50 ml (2 fl oz) fresh orange juice

Trim the rhubarb and cut the stalks into short lengths. Put into a greased 900 ml (1½ pint) ovenproof dish. Mix the breadcrumbs, sugar and ginger together and sprinkle over the rhubarb. Spoon the orange juice gently over the crumbs. Bake in the oven at Gas Mark 3 (160°C, 325°F) for 40 minutes or until the fruit is soft and the topping browned. Serve hot or cold.

## Carrot and Date Cake

MAKES APPROXIMATELY 16 SLICES

50 g (2 oz) polyunsaturated margarine
6 tbsp honey
¼ tsp sunflower oil
100 g (4 oz) carrots, peeled
100 g (4 oz) dates, stoned
175 g (6 oz) plain granary flour
1 level tsp bicarbonate of soda
½ level tsp baking powder
½ level tsp cinnamon
1 egg
120 ml (4 fl oz) skimmed milk
3 tbsp unsweetened orange juice

Line a 15 cm (6 inch) square tin with greaseproof paper and brush with a little oil.

Place the margarine and honey in a small pan and warm until it has melted. Finely grate the carrots and chop the dates.

Mix together the flour, bicarbonate of soda, baking powder and cinnamon.

Beat the egg with the milk and orange juice until blended. Add the egg mixture to the honey and margarine mixture. Stir all the ingredients together gently until thoroughly mixed. Pour the mixture into the tin and bake in a preheated oven at Gas Mark 5 (190°C, 375°F) for one hour. Place on a wire rack and leave to cool.

# Long-term lifestyle

## _____ Natalie's story _____

Natalie is a 34-year-old legal secretary, who is married and lives in London. She had previously consulted the WNAS for her severe PMS some six years ago, and had been extremely well until a year ago, when she developed IBS.

'I was feeling so well after following the WNAS programme in 1987, so much so that I drifted back to some of my old eating habits thinking that I could get away with it. I developed constipation and severe abdominal bloating with pain, which got progressively worse over a period of a year.

'My doctor diagnosed IBS, and because I was having indigestion and burning as well, I was sent for an endoscopy. This only found that I was producing considerable bile. My stomach used to blow up and become hard and heavy, like a cannon ball. On one occasion I had to be sent home from work, and on another I was in such pain – I couldn't even stand up – that I had to lie down.

'I went back to the WNAS clinic in London for a review appointment. After not drinking coffee for a long time, I had gradually begun to drink several cups each day. Since stopping the coffee again the symptoms have gone. Once again I am staggered at the power of diet on my body. It has taught me that in order to remain healthy, and symptom free, I cannot deviate too far from the diet.'

---

Once Phase 8 is complete, you should have reached some firm conclusions about your diet in relation to your symptoms. In an ideal world you should be symptom free and aware of the foods and drinks that trigger your problems. There may however be a few grey areas, in which case you may need to do a bit more detective work over the next few weeks. If you remain unsure about certain aspects of your diet, cut them out again for a few days, and then re-introduce them one by one, leaving three or four days in between each item. Once again you will need to chart your findings carefully, so that you can review your progress and see clear results.

When you have been symptom free for several months, you may feel like trying some of the foods or drinks that you reacted to. Err on the cautious side, and only try suspect foods or drinks when you have a quiet few days and, if you are a menstruating female, make sure the trial does not take place in your premenstrual phase. If once again you get a reaction, you will have to continue to avoid those aspects of your diet and use alternatives. If you seem to be all right with the former suspect substances, then include them in small amounts in your diet until you are sure.

As a general rule, it is recommended that you try out most of the foods that you have reacted adversely to every two to three months. If you keep having problems with these food groups after six months then the following long-term pointers will apply.

# Alternative foods and drinks

Once you have identified the food groups that trigger your symptoms, you will need to look for alternatives for the long term. Let us look at each group of food in the order they arise in the Plan.

## *Potato and corn*

This group is not too difficult to replace. You can get your starch from fruit, vegetables – especially other root vegetables, rice, buckwheat, millet, wheat, oats, barley and rye if they are tolerated. You may be able to improve your tolerance to corn if you cook it well and chew it thoroughly, or if it is processed or ground as in corn flakes or cornflour.

## *Citrus fruits*

Again this group is not too hard to do without. There are plenty of other fruits and fruit juices to choose from. You would have to be very sensitive to lemons not to be able to tolerate the odd squirt of lemon juice in a recipe, or a slice of lemon in a drink. Also it has been our experience that very fresh and tangy citrus fruits may be more likely to cause problems than those that have aged a little when their skin is beginning to wrinkle. In the summer a glass of orange or other citrus fruit juice can quickly deteriorate and the fermentation that takes place can cause bowel problems. This is not necessarily due to the citrus content but to acids and other products of fermentation.

Finally, citric acid, one of the many natural chemicals in citrus fruit, is often added to foods as an acidifying agent, for example in some canned drinks. While some people react to this, it is by no means the rule that being sensitive to citrus fruit automatically means that you will react to citric acid. It is all a matter of trial and error.

## Dairy products

Reactions to cow's milk are quite common and do have a reputation for being long lasting. If the reaction to lactose (milk sugar) is diarrhoea, this may be temporary following a stomach infection, and it may improve after a course of strong vitamin B supplements. Hard cheese has relatively little lactose and so may be tolerated, and semi-skimmed or fully skimmed milk may also be acceptable to a minority of people who cannot tolerate full fat milk. It is worth a try.

Apart from this, other reactions to cow's milk are most likely to be due to reactions to the protein component, which can also on occasion cause eczema, asthma and rhinitis – a running or watery nose and headaches. Some people who react to cow's milk can tolerate sheep's or goat's milk, but probably no more than 50 per cent. A small percentage can also tolerate condensed milk but this is rare. Very often this type of reaction does mean long-term avoidance of cow's milk and with this a fall in the dietary intake of calcium.

Fortunately, there are a wide variety of soya products including milks, yoghurts and ice creams, many of which are fortified with extra calcium. Most supermarkets sell soya milk, often sweetened with fructose. It can be used in the same way as ordinary milk, in drinks and for cereals. Soya yoghurts are also available and can be used in sauces and dips. Many manufacturers now produce soya ice cream, which is often so similar to the cow's milk varieties that you can hardly notice the difference. The favourite is a brand called Tuti, which is available in health food shops, and Berrydales also make a whole range.

Daily long-term calcium supplements should be considered for all those who cannot take dairy products especially the elderly, pregnant and breastfeeding women, women at the time of the menopause, those who are physically inactive and children. This is worth discussing with your doctor because calcium supplements of 400-1000 mg are available on the National Health Service.

## *Yeast rich foods*

This mixed and varied group includes yeast extract, many savoury snacks, gravy, most bought soups, vinegar, pickles and most alcoholic beverages. Reactions can be varied and once again a fair amount of trial and error is necessary. For example, some people may react to alcohol but not to Marmite, some to wine and beer but not lager. If you do find that you get a reaction to alcohol, it may be worth trying gin and vodka as they are more likely to be tolerated. Bear in mind that wine contains not only alcohol and yeast but often sulphite, as a preservative, which can contribute to the formation of bad-eggs gas. If you are really yeast sensitive, it is unlikely that you will even be able to tolerate low-alcohol wines or beer either.

Lemon juice is fortunately a good substitute for vinegar, but you will need to avoid eating pickled foods. There are some gravy preparations that do not contain yeast. They can be found in some health food shops.

## *Wheat, oats, barley and rye*

These four cereals all contain gluten, and quite a lot about their long-term avoidance can be found in a number of books on gluten-free cooking. You may think that the prospect of life without these staples is pretty dim, but do not forget that large parts of China, Southern India, and South-East Asia live with rice as their main cereal, and with little or none of these gluten-containing grains. Many of these groups do not have cow's milk either. So such diets are possible, healthy and enjoyable.

There is an important point here about those with apparent intolerance to these grains. A severe form of allergy to these foods occurs in the condition coeliac disease. The symptoms are similar to IBS but in addition there is loss of weight, anaemia, nutritional deficiencies or other health problems. This diagnosis should be considered in anyone with these features who repeatedly reacts to gluten-containing cereals. You will need to pay a visit to your doctor if you think that this may apply to you. If you prove to have severe gluten sensitivity then certain gluten-free foods can be prescribed under the National Health Service. This is not the case for those who simply have IBS and an intolerance to wheat.

If it happens to be wheat, oats, barley and rye that you find hard to tolerate, you will need to use other grains as substitutes. Bread can be made from rice and potato flour, or buckwheat and potato flour.

There are many varieties of rice noodles, available from Chinese supermarkets, which are a good reasonably priced substitute for pasta. You will also find rice, corn and buckwheat pasta available in health food shops.

Your local pharmacist is usually a good source of alternative products, and they usually keep a stock for their customers with coeliac disease. They will be able to order biscuits, cakes, crackers and bread for you, although they can be expensive. Glutafin make a good range of cakes, biscuits and crackers and EnergG do good rice breads. The Mexican shelf at supermarkets usually has a good stock of corn products, which can be incorporated into meals or used as snacks with dips.

There are many flours available for cooking. You can make almost anything from cakes to pancakes using flour made from corn, rice, buckwheat, potato, dal and cassava. Cakes and biscuits can be baked successfully with a combination of ground nuts and rice, corn or potato flour. When making pastry with alternative flours, it is best to roll it out on to baking paper, as it tends to stick to the work-surface. Once it has reached the size required, you simply turn it over into the dish.

Sometimes wholewheat causes a reaction, but white flour, or oats, barley and rye may be acceptable. You will need to determine which suits your gut in the medium and long term. French bread, made with French flour, which most supermarkets now stock, has a lower gluten content. If you react to flour, it may be worth trying this variety to see whether it can be tolerated. Some patients manage well with rye and are able to eat rye crackers regularly, while others can manage with oats, and use oat cereals, Jordan's Frusli bars and flapjacks without any ill effects.

As wheat, oats, barley and rye provide us with important amounts of fibre, it is important to eat extra fruit and vegetable fibre in order to make up for the loss. Also, ensure you have a good intake of dairy products to make up the calcium shortfall, and if dairy products are off your menu, then you will almost certainly need to speak to your doctor about obtaining some calcium supplements.

# What is wrong with some missing favourites?

At the end of the Plan you will undoubtedly have noticed that there are certain dietary items that you may not have had the opportunity to try out or add back. They include tea, coffee, cola and other soft drinks, sugar, sweets and chocolate. This is as good a place as any to say a few words about them, as you will probably want to re-introduce some of them.

## *Tea*

The main reason for avoiding tea in the long term is if you suffer with constipation, which tea can aggravate. You may be able to get away with two or three weak cups a day without any ill effects. Because of its caffeine content, tea should also be limited if you suffer with anxiety problems or insomnia. The high tannin content of tea is relevant to vegetarians as it greatly impedes the absorption of iron from vegetarian protein, which is especially relevant to menstruating and pregnant women and the elderly of both sexes.

## *Coffee*

Diarrhoea can be aggravated by coffee, and if you have a nervous disposition, you should avoid coffee because of its caffeine content. Like tea, high intakes of coffee can also interfere with the absorption of iron and other minerals.

## *Soft drinks*

Cola-based drinks usually contain caffeine and are therefore best avoided. Ordinary canned drinks are high in sugar and phosphates. Consumption of sugar in Western communities is approximately twice the level that is considered desirable for good health, so we are not about to recommend that you consume anything other than the occasional drink of these. A deficiency of phosphorus is virtually unknown as it is widely distributed in almost all foods, good and bad.

## Alternatives to caffeine-based drinks

If tea and coffee aggravate your symptoms, you will need to find alternatives that you feel happy with, and you will find that there are many to choose from. You may like to try some of the decaffeinated varieties of tea and coffee, but restrict your intake to no more than three or four cups a day. Rooibosch Eleven O'clock herbal tea is a very acceptable ordinary tea look-alike. It is a caffeine-free, low tannin tea bag that can be made with or without milk. It also contains a natural muscle relaxant, and so may be very useful if you suffer with abdominal spasms. It is available from most health food shops. There are now so many different varieties of herbal fruit teas, most of which come in single trial sachets, that if you persevere you will undoubtedly find one or two that appeal.

If you have a problem with grains you will be restricted to dandelion coffee or chicory as coffee substitutes. Dandelion coffee comes in two varieties, instant, which is pretty sweet, and dandelion root, which when boiled up, or put through a 'coffee' filter makes a very nice strong brew, with or without milk. If you manage well with barley and rye, there are a number of coffee substitutes that you can try which are cereal based. Barley Cup is the favourite cereal-based drink, which comes in coffee-coloured powder form and is available from health food shops. Other varieties to try are Bambu and Caro.

These days, there are many healthy varieties of carbonated drinks to choose from. Fizzy bottled water with or without fruit juice is about the most basic and inexpensive. Appletise, a fizzy apple juice, is widely available, as is Citrus Spring, a spring water and citrus drink, which is fine as long as you can tolerate citrus. These are just a few of the varieties available from supermarkets and garages alike. Just remember to read the labels before you try something new.

## *Sugar and sweets*

Expert committees advise that we should all reduce our sugar consumption by approximately half. Dental decay is strongly linked to sugar consumption and reduction in intake is often needed if you are overweight, or suffer with diabetes, gall stones, kidney stones, high levels of blood cholesterol or other fats. Very occasionally sucrose intolerance occurs, and as a result of consuming even small amounts of sugar can cause abdominal discomfort and diarrhoea. This is a rare condition, which is usually hereditary.

Many sweets contain artificial colourings in addition to sugar, which can trigger eczema, asthma, rhinitis, and overactive behaviour in young children.

## *Chocolate*

Though chocolate is an excellent trigger for migraine headaches and sometimes eczema, only rarely does it seem to aggravate IBS symptoms. It is, however, high in sugar, fat and calories. Milk chocolate may not be tolerated if you are sensitive to cow's milk or lactose, and many chocolate bars have a wheat biscuit base and contain nuts, raisins and other ingredients. Once again you will need to read the labels carefully.

### Sweet alternatives

If sugar and chocolate upset your gut, you will need to do without or substitute them with sweet snacks. Dried fruits are very sweet, and can be eaten freely, as long as you do not have a problem with yeast-based foods. Most health food shops sell a range of dried fruit bars, and packets of dried fruit sweets. Granovita fruit bars are particularly delicious, as are little dried fruit 'sweets' called 'La Fruit', made by Lyme Regis Foods. Many fresh fruits are sweet, and when combined with nuts or seeds make a very satisfying and nutritious snack.

If sugar itself causes you problems, try using fructose in your cooking. Dietade make a product called 'Fruit Sugar' which comes in a packet and can be purchased in most health food shops and supermarkets. As it is almost twice as sweet as ordinary sugar, you will only need to use half the amount stated for sugar when following a recipe. Combined with nuts, eggs and alternative flours if necessary, you can use it for very acceptable biscuits and cakes.

Sadly, there is no real alternative to chocolate. Green & Black's dark chocolate, available in most health foodshops and some supermarkets, is about the most wholesome, and we think it is delicious. Some people eat carob bars instead of chocolate and find them acceptable, while others prefer to do without. Making sure you have some acceptable desserts to follow your meals and some wholesome cakes and biscuits handy for snacks does help to keep the cravings for chocolate at bay.

# To cheat or not to cheat?

As our memory of pain dulls with time, once you have been symptom free for a while, you may well be tempted to veer off the straight and narrow nutritional path. If it is any consolation, you will not be the first or the last to do so. As we said earlier, this is only human nature. If your symptoms return each time you break your diet, you will reach an inevitable point where you have to decide whether you prefer to live without the symptoms or without the food or drink in question. It is sometimes a straight trade off, and only you can make the final decision. If the symptoms are minor, you may decide the occasional indulgence is worth it. However, if the indulgence takes you back to square one, you may decide that you prefer your good health.

Most of our ex-patients get addicted to good health and wouldn't seriously go back to the foods and drinks that they know upset them in the long term. They have all been surprised at how enjoyable a 'restricted' diet can be, and amazed at the variety of new foods and drinks available as alternatives.

Our advice to you is to follow the ten-week plan methodically, while keeping your short-term expectations conservative. Keep accurate records, so that you can spot the offending foods at a glance, and don't get disheartened if you do get a reaction. Make plenty of time for rest, relaxation and exercise, and brief your family and friends so that they can support you while you are conducting the experiment. We think you will be pleasantly pleased with the results, and would very much like to hear about your success.

If you feel that you need extra help to get started, or would like some expert monitoring, the WNAS have clinics and a postal telephone consultation line which you can use. The WNAS details are listed on page 247.

We very much hope that by following the recommendations that we have set out, you will manage to overcome your IBS symptoms, and as a result live a long and healthy life.

# Appendix

## Recommended Reading List
NOTE: UK, US and A denote the following books are available in Great Britain, the United States and Australia.

### General

*Every Woman's Health Guide* by Maryon Stewart and Dr Alan Stewart, Headline. **UK A**

*How to Stop Smoking and Stay Stopped for Good* by Gillian Riley, Vermilion. **UK**

*Getting Sober and Loving It* by Joan and Derek Taylor, Vermilion (out of print). **UK**

*Coming Off Tranquillizers and Sleeping Pills* by Dr Susan Trickett, Thorsons. **UK USA A** (Lothian Publishing Co).

*The Book of Massage* by Lucy Lidell, Ebury Press. **UK**

*Do-it-yourself Shiatsu* by W. Ohashi, Unwin Hyman (out of print). **UK**

*Nutritional Medicine* by Dr Stephen Davies and Dr Alan Stewart, Pan Books. **UK A**

*The Y Plan Countdown*, Hamlyn. **UK**

*The Book of Yoga*, by The Sivananda Yoga Centre, Ebury Press. **UK A**

*Aromatherapy* by Gill Martin, Vermilion. **UK**

*Alternative Health Osteopathy* by Stephen Sandler, Optima (out of print). **UK**

*Acupuncture* by Martin Nightingale, Vermilion. **UK**

*Bone Boosters - Natural Ways to Beat Osteoporosis* by Diana Moran and Helen-Franks, Boxtree. **UK**

*Escape from Tranquillizers Band Sleeping Pills* by Larry Nield, Ebury Press. **UK**

*The Women's Guide to Homoeopathy* by Dr Andrew Lockie and Dr Nicola Geddes, Hamish Hamilton. **UK**

*Natural Hormone Health* by Arabella Melville, Thorsons. **UK**

*Alexander Technique* by Chris Stevens, Random House.

*Homeopathy for the First Aider* by Dorothy Shepherd, The C.W. Daniel Co. Ltd. **UK USA**

*Evening Primrose Oil* by Judy Graham, Thorsons.

*Aromatherapy for Women and Children* by Jane Dye, The C.W. Daniel Co. Ltd. **UK USA**

*A Guide to Herbal Remedies* by Mark Evans, The C.W. Daniel Co. Ltd. **UK USA**

### Stress

*Self Help for your Nerves* by Dr Clair Weekes, Thorsons. **UK USA** (Hawthorne Publishing Co.)

*Stress and Relaxation Self-help Techniques for Everyone* by Jane Madden, Optima. **UK USA A**

*Lyn Marshall's Instant Stress Cure* by Lyn Marshall, Vermilion. **UK A**

*Stress Wise* by Dr Terry Looker and Dr Olga Gregson, Headway. **UK**

*Tranquillization: BThe Non-Addictive Way* by Phyllis Speight, The C.W. Daniel Co. Ltd. **UK USA**

## Diet

*The New Why You Don't Need Meat* by Peter Cox, Bloomsbury. **UK A**
*The Allergy Diet* by Elizabeth Workman SRD, Dr John Hunter and Virginia Alun Jones, Martin Dunitz. **UK USA**
*The Food Intolerance Diet* by Elizabeth Workman SRD, Dr John Hunter and Dr Virginia Alun Jones, Vermilion. **UK USA**
*Food Allergy and Intolerance* by Jonathan Brostoff and Linda Gamlin, Bloomsbury. **UK A**
*The Salt-free Diet Book* by Dr Graham McGregor, Optima (out of print). **UK USA**
*Organic Consumer Guide: Food You Can Trust* edited by David Mabey and Alan and Jackie Gear, Thorsons. **UK**
*Food Irradiation: The Facts* by Tony Webb and Dr Tim Lang, Thorsons. **UK**
*Food Allergy and Intolerance* by Jonathan Bristoff and Linda Gamlin, Bloomsbury. **UK A**

## Recipe Books

*Good Food Gluten Free* by Hilda Cherry Hills, Keats. **USA**
*Gluten-Free Cookery* by Rita Greer, Thorsons. **UK**
*The Wheat and Gluten Free Cookbook* by Joan Noble, Vermilion. **UK A**
*The Candida Albicans Yeast-Free Cook Book* by Pat Connolly and Associates of the Price Pottinger Nutrition Foundation, Keats. UK USA
*The Cranks Recipe Book* by David Canter, Hay Canter and Daphne Swann, Orion. **UK**
*Raw Energy Recipes* by Leslie and Susannah Kenton, Century. **UK**
*The Reluctant Vegetarian Cookbook* by Simon Hope, Heinemann. **UK**
*Gourmet Vegetarian Cooking* by Rose Elliot, Thorsons. **UK A**
*The Gluten-free and Wheat-free Bumper Bake Book* by Rita Greer, Bunterbird Ltd. **UK**
*The Single Vegan* by Leah Leneman, Thorsons.
*Whole Earth Cookbook* by Hilary Meth, Vermilion. **UK**

## Exercise

Diana Moran's 3 in 1 Workout video by Diana Moran.
*The Ys Way to Physical Fitness* by Clayton R Myers and Lawrence A Golding (available from YMCA, see page 243).
*YMCA Guide to Exercise Music* by RodneyCullum and Leslie Mowbray (available from YMCA, see page 243).

## Useful Addresses

AAA (Action Against Allergy)
PO Box 278, Twickenham TW1 42Q

Al-Anon Family Groups
61 Great Dover Street, London SE1 4YF
Tel: 0171 403 0888

Alcohol Concern
Waterbridge House, 32-36 Lomar Street, London SE1 0EE
Tel: 0181 767 1827

Alcoholics Anonymous (AA)
General Services Office, PO Box 1, Stonebow House, York YO1 2NJ
Tel: 01904 644026

Allergycare
Pollards Yard, Wood Street, Taunton, Somerset TA1 1UP
Tel: 01823 325023

Anorexia & Bulimia Care
15 Fernhurst Gate, Aughton, Ormskirk, Lancashire L39 5EP
Tel: 01695 422479

ASH -The Campaign for Freedom From Tobacco
Devon House, 12-15 Dartmouth Street, London SW1H 9BL
Tel: 0171 314 1360

British Acupuncture Register and Directory
34 Alderney Street, London SW1V 4EU
Tel: 0171 834 1012

British Association for Counselling
1 Regent Place, Rugby, Warwickshire CV21 2PJ
Tel: 01788 578328 (info)

British Homeopathic Association
27A Devonshire Street, London W1N 1RJ
Tel: 0171 935 2163

British Hypnotherapy Association
67 Upper Berkeley Street, London W1H 7DH
Tel: 0171 723 4443

British Society for Allergy and Clinical Immunology
66 Western Park, Thames Ditton, Surrey KT7 0HL
Fax: 0181 398 2766

British Society of Allergy and Environmental Medicine
'Acorns', Ramsey Road, Cadnam, Southampton SO4 2NN
Tel: 01713 812124

British Wheel of Yoga
1 Hamilton Place, Boston Road, Sleaford,Lincolnshire NG34 7ES
Tel: 01529 306851

Chiropractic Patients Association
8 Centre One, Lysander Way, Old Sarum Park, Salisbury, Wiltshire SP4 6BU
Tel: 01722 416027

Coeliac Society
PO Box 220, High Wycombe, Buckinghamshire HP11 2HY
Tel: 01494 37278

College of Health
St Margarets House, 21 Old Ford Road, London E2 9PL
Tel: 0181 9831225

College of Traditional Chinese Acupuncture
Tao House, Queensway, Leamington Spa, Warwickshire CV32 5EZ
Tel: 01926 393347

Depression Alliance
35 Westminster Bridge Road, London SE1 7JB
Tel: 0171 633 9929

Eating Disorders Association
Sackville Place, 44 Magdalen Street, Norwich NR3 1JU
Tel: 01603 621414

Friends of the Earth
26-28 Underwood Street, London N1 7JQ
Tel: 0171 490 1555

IBS Network/Gut Reaction Centre for Human Nutrition
Northern General Hospital, Sheffield S5 7AU

National Association for Colitis and Crohns Disease
PO Box 205, St Albans, Hertfordshire AL1 1AB
Tel: 01727 844296

National Back Pain Association
31-33 Park Road,Teddington, Middlesex TW11 0AB
Tel: 0181 977 5474/5

National Federation of Spiritual Healers
Old Manor Farm Studio, Church Street, Sunbury-on-Thames, Middlesex TW16 6RG
Tel: 01932 783164/5

National Institute of Medical Herbalists
56 Longbrook Street, Exeter, Devon EX4 6AH
Tel: 01392 426022

National Society for Research into Allergy
PO Box 45, Hinckley, Leicestershire LE10 1JY
Tel: 01455 851546

Samaritans
10 The Grove, Slough SL1 1QP
Tel: 01753 532713

Shiatsu Society
31 Pullman Lane, Godalming, Surrey GU7 1XY
Tel: 01483 860771

The British Acupuncture Council
Park House, 206-208 Latimer Road, London W10 2RE
Tel: 0181 964 0222

The British School of Osteopathy
1-4 Suffolk Street, London, SW1 4HG
Tel: 0171 930 9254

The Exercise Association
Unit 4, Angel Gate, City Road, London EC1V 2PT
Tel: 0171 278 0811

The Faculty of Homeopathy
Hannemann House, 2 Powis Place, Great Ormond Street, London WC1N 3HT
Tel: 0171 837 9469

The Henry Doubleday Research Association
Ryton Organic Gardens, Ryton on Dunsmore, Coventry CV8 3LG
Tel: 01203 303517

The Sports Council
16 Upper Woburn Place, London WC1H 0QP
Tel: 0171 388 1277

Tranx Release (Northampton)
81 St Giles Street, Northampton NN1 1JF
Tel: 01604 22121

UK College for Complementary Healthcare Studies
St Charles Hospital, Exmoor Street, London W10 6D2
Tel: 0181 964 1206

Vegan Society
Donald Watson House, 7 Battle Road, St Leonards-on-Sea, East Sussex TN3Y 7AA
Tel: 01424 427393

Vegetarian Society
Parkdale, Dunham Road, Altrincham, Cheshire WA14 4QG
Tel: 0161 928 0793

Womens Nutritional Advisory Service
PO Box 268, Lewes, East Sussex BN7 2QN
Tel: 01273 487366

YMCA
112 Great Russell Street, London WC1B 3NQ
Tel: 0171 637 8131

Yoga for Health Foundation
Ickwell Bury, Biggleswade, Bedfordshire SG18 9EF
Tel: 01767 627271

## Stockists

*Efamol Evening Primrose Oil*
Chemists, health food shops and Nutritional Health (mail order)
**\*Mail Order Address**
Nutritional Health Limited
PO Box 926, Lewes, East Sussex BN7 2QL.

*Heat pads*
Nutritional Health (mail order)\*.

*Linusit Gold*
Health food shops.

*Magnesium Amino Acid Chelate*
Nutritional Health (mail order)\*.

*Optivite*
Boots, health food shops and Nutritional Health (mail order)\*.

# References

## Chapters 1 and 2

1 Connell A.M., Hilton C., Irvine G. et al. Variation of bowel habit in two population samples. British Medical Journal. 1965;2:1095-1099.
2 Drossman D.A., Sandler R.S., McKee D.C., Lovitz A.J. Bowel patterns among subjects not seeking health care. Gastroenterology 1982;83:529-534.
3 Heaton K. W., O'Donnell L. J. D., Braddon F. E. M., Mountford R. A., Hughes A. O., Cripps P. J. Gastroenterology 1992;102:1962-1967.
4 Danivat D., Tankeyoon M., Sritratanaban A. Prevalence of irritable bowel syndrome in a non-Western population. British Medical Journal. 1988;296:17105.
5 Jones R., Lydeard S. Irritable bowel syndrome in the general population. British Medical Journal. 1992;304:87-90.
6 Isgar B., Harman M., Kaye M. D., Whorwell P. J. Symptoms of irritable bowel syndrome in ulcerative colitis in remission. Gut. 1983;24:190-192.
7 Whitehead W.E., Crowell M. D., Robinson J. C., Heller B. R., Schuster M. M. Effects of stressful life events on bowel symptoms: subjects with irritable bowel syndrome compared with subjects without bowel dysfunction. Gut. 1992;33:825-830.
8 Thompson W. G. Irritable bowel syndrome: pathogenesis and management. The Lancet. 1993;341:1569-1572.
9 Waller S. L. Misiewicz J. J. Prognosis in the irritable bowel syndrome: a prospective study. The Lancet. 1969;2:753-756.
10 Chaudhary N.A., Truelove S. C. The irritable colon syndrome. Quarterly Journal of Medicine. 1962; 31: 307-32.
11 Harvey R. F., Mauad E. C., Brown A. M. Prognosis in the irritable bowel syndrome: a 5-year prospective study. The Lancet. 1987;1:963-965.
12 Faussone Pellegrini M.S., Ibba Manneschi L., Manneschi L. The caecocolonic junction in humans has a sphincteric anatomy and function. Gut. 1995;37:493-498.
13 Gwee K. A., Read N. W., et al. Psychometric scores and persistence of irritable bowel after infectious diarrhoea. The Lancet, 1996;347:150-153.

## Chapter 3 – symptoms

1 Maxton D. G., Morris J. A., Whorwell P. J. Ranking of symptoms by patients with irritable bowel syndrome. British Medical Journal. 1989;299:1138.
2 Manning A. P., Thompson W. G., Heaton K. W., Morris A. F. Towards positive diagnosis of the irritable bowel. British Medical Journal. 1978;2:653-654.
3 O'Donnell L. J. D., Virjee J., Heaton K. W. Detection of pseudodiarrhoea by simple clinical assessment of intestinal transit rate. British Medical Journal. 1990;300:439-440.
4 Whorwell P.J., McCallum M., Creed F. H., Roberts C. T. Non-colonic features of irritable bowel syndrome. Gut 1986;27:37-40.
5 Jones R., Lydeard S. Irritable bowel syndrome in the general population. British Medical Journal. 1992;304:87-90.
6 Thompson W. G. Irritable bowel syndrome: pathogenesis and management. The Lancet. 1993;341:1569-1572.

## Chapter 5 – constipation

1 Editorial. Constipation in young women. The Lancet. 1986;1:778-779.
2 Petrakis N. L., King E. B. Cytological abnormalities in nipple aspirates of breast fluid from women with severe constipation. The Lancet. 1981;2:1203-1205.

3 Turnbull G. K., Lennard-Jones J. E., Bartram C. I. Failure of rectal expulsion as a cause of constipation: why fibre and laxatives sometimes fail. The Lancet. 1986;1767-769.

4 Preston D.M., Lennard-Jones J. E. Severe chronic constipation of young women: 'idiopathic slow transit constipation'. Gut. 1986;27:41-48.

5 Heaton J.W., Oettle G.J. Bowel symptoms and the pelvic floor. The Lancet. 1986;1:1207.

6 Stephen A. M. Should we eat more fibre? Journal of Human Nutrition. 1981;35:403-414.

7 Manning A. P., Heaton K. W., Harvey R. F., Uglow P. Wheat fibre and irritable bowel syndrome. The Lancet. 1977;2:417-418.

8 Cann P. A., Read N. W., Holdsworth C. D. What is the benefit of wheat bran in patients with irritable bowel syndrome? Gut. 1984;25:168-173.

9 Alun Jones V., McLaughlan P., Shorthouse M., Workman E., Hunter J. O. Food intolerance: a major factor in the pathogenesis of irritable bowel syndrome. The Lancet. 1982;2:1115-1117.
   Also Letter. Food intolerance and irritable bowel syndrome. The Lancet. 1983;2:633-64.

10 Morley J. E. et al. Effect of exorphins on gastrointestinal function, hormonal release, and appetite. Gastroenterology. 1983;84:1517-1523.

11 Kumar D., Wingate D. L. The irritable bowel syndrome: a paroxysmal motor disorder. The Lancet. 1985;2:973-977.

12 Taylor R. Management of constipation. British Medical Journal. 1990;300:1063-1065.

13 Spiller R. When fibre fails. British Medical Journal 1990;300:1065-1067.

14 Hojgaard L., Arffmann S., Jorgensen M., Kragg E. Tea consumption a cause of constipation. British Medical Journal 1981;282:864.

15 Sherwood R. S., Rocks B., Stewart A. Saxton. Magnesium and the premenstrual syndrome. Annals of Clinical Biochemistry. 1986;23:667-670.

16 Cotterell J.C., Lee A. J., Hunter J. O. Double-blind cross-over trial of evening primrose oil in women with menstrually related irritable bowel syndrome. Also, Omega-6 Essential Fatty Acids, pp421-426. Edited by Horrobin D. F.; published by Wiley-Liss. New York. 1990.

17 Alun Jones V. The irritable bowel syndrome. Food and the Gut, pp208-220. Edited by Hunter J. O. and Alun Jones V.; published by Balliere Tindall. London. 1985.

## Chapter 6 – diarrhoea

1 Report by the Royal College of Physicians. 1984: Food Allergy and Intolerance.

2 Cooper B. T., Holmes G. K. T., Ferguson R. A., Thompson R. N. A., Cooke W. T. Gluten-sensitive diarrhoea without evidence of coeliac disease. Gastroenterology. 1980;79:801-806.

3 Arnason J. A., Gudjonsson H., Freysdottir J., Jonsdottir I., Valdimarsson H. Do adults with high gliadin antibody concentrations have subclinical gluten intolerance? Gut. 1992;33:194-197.

4 Editorial. Milk fat, diarrhoea and the ileal brake. The Lancet. 1986;2:658.

5 Editorial. Hastening Gut Transit. The Lancet. 1990;2:974.

6 Banerjee A. K. Enteropathy induced by non-steroidal anti-inflammatory drugs. British Medical Journal. 1989;298:1539-1540.

7 Merliss R. R., Hofman A. Steatorrhoea following the use of antibiotics. The New England Journal of Medicine. 1951;245:328-330.

8 Vazquez-Olivencia W., Shah P., Pitchumoni C. S. The effect of red and black pepper on orocaecal transit time. Journal of the American College of Nutrition. 1992;11:228-234.
9 Bennett J. R. Progress report: Smoking and the gastrointestinal tract. Gut. 1972;13:658-665.
10 Fine K. D., Fordtran J. S. The effect of diarrhoea on fecal fat excretion. Gastroenterology. 1992;102:1936-1939.
11 Moriarty K. J. The irritable bowel syndrome. British Medical Journal. 1992;304:1166-1169.
12 Bolin T. D. Use of oral sodium cromoglycate in persistent diarrhoea. Gut. 1980;21:848-850.
13 Report of the Royal College of Physicians and the British Nutrition Foundation. Food Intolerance and Food Aversion. RCP Publications. 1984. London.
14 Ladas S. D., Haritos D. N., Raptis S. A. Honey may have a laxative effect on normal subjects because of incomplete fructose absorption. American Journal of Clinical Nutrition. 1995;62:1212-1215.
15 Hoekstra J. H., van den Aker J. H. L., Hartemink R., Kneepkens C. M. F. Fruit juice malabsorption: not only fructose. Acta Paediatrica 1995;84:1241-1244.
16 McLeod John R., Bennett H. P. J., Hamilton J. R. Inhibition of intestinal secretion by rice. The Lancet. 1995;246:909-992.

## *Chapter 7 – pain*

1 Editorial. Balloons in the irritable bowel. The Lancet. 1985;2:427-428.
2 Trotman I. F., Price C. C. Bloated irritable bowel syndrome defined by dynamic 99mTc bran scan. The Lancet. 1986;2:364-366.
3 Thompson W. G. Irritable bowl syndrome: pathogenesis and management. The Lancet.1993;1:1569-1572.
4 Chambers J. B., Bland J. M. Hyperventilation and the irritable bowel syndrome. The Lancet. 1986;1:221.

## *Chapter 8 – wind and bloating*

1 Maxton D. G., Martin D. F., Whorwell P. J., Godfrey M. Abdominal distension in female patients with irritable bowel syndrome: exploration of possible mechanisms. Gut. 1991;32:62-64.
2 Cummings J. H. Fermentation in the human large intestine: evidence and implications for health. The Lancet. 1983;1:1206-1209.
3 Hunter J. O. Food allergy – or enterometabolic disorder? The Lancet. 1991;2:495-496.
4 Calloway S. P., Fonagy P. Aerophagia and irritable bowel syndrome. The Lancet. 1985;2:1368.
5 Levitt M. D., Lasser R. N., Schwartz J. S., Bond J. H. Studies of a flatulent patient. The New England Journal of Medicine. 1976; 295:260-262.
6 Editorial. The colon, the rumen, and d-lactic acidosis. The Lancet. 1990;336:599-600.
7 Trotman I. F., Price C. C. Bloated irritable bowel syndrome defined by dynamic 99mTc bran scan. The Lancet. 1986;2:364-366.
8 Christl S. U., Gibson G. R., Cummings J. H. Role of dietary sulphate in the regulation of methanogenesis in the human large intestine. Gut. 1992;33:1234-1238.

## *Chapter 10 – stress*

1 Swedlund J., Sjoden L., Ottosson J. O., Doteval G. Controlled study of psychological treatment for the irritable bowel syndrome. The Lancet. 1983;2:589-591.

2  Guthrie E., Creed F., Dawson D., Tomenson B. A controlled trial of psychological treatment for the irritable bowel syndrome. Gastroenterology.
   1991;100:450-457.
3  Whorwell P. J., Prior A., Colgan S. M. Hypnotherapy in severe irritable bowel
   syndrome: further experience. Gut. 1987;28:423-425.
4  Harvey R. F., Hinton R. A., Gunary R. M., Barry R. E. Individual and group
   hypnotherapy in the treatment of refractory irritable bowel syndrome. The
   Lancet. 1989;1:424-425.

## Further Help

For further information, please send a large self-addressed envelope plus four
separate 1st class stamps to the Woman's Nutritional Advisory Service, PO BOX
268, Lewes, East Sussex BN7 2QN.

## Advice Lines from the WNAS

| | |
|---|---|
| OVERCOME PMS NATURALLY | 0839 556600 |
| THE PMS DIET LINE | 0839 556601 |
| OVERCOME MENOPAUSE NATURALLY | 0839 556602 |
| THE MENOPAUSE DIET LINE | 0839 556603 |
| BEAT SUGAR CRAVING | 0839 556604 |
| THE VITALITY DIET LINE | 0839 556605 |
| OVERCOMING BREAST TENDERNESS | 0839 556606 |
| OVERCOME PERIOD PAINS NATURALLY | 0839 556607 |
| GET FIT FOR PREGNANCY AND BREASTFEEDING | 0839 556608 |
| SKIN, NAIL & HAIR SIGNS OF DEFICIENCY | 0839 556609 |
| IMPROVE LIBIDO NATURALLY | 0839 556610 |
| BEAT IRRITABLE BOWEL SYNDROME | 0839 556611 |
| OVERCOME FATIGUE | 0839 556612 |
| BEAT MIGRAINE NATURALLY | 0839 556613 |
| OVERCOME OVULATION PAIN | 0839 556614 |
| DIRECTORY | 0839 556615 |

# Index